ENDORSEMENTS

"*Rise Above It* fills readers with hope while inspiring them to make a commitment to life! It is a must read with such a powerful message for all students and leaders alike."

Robin Jones
Principal of Chief Ivan Blunka School in New Stuyahok, Alaska
2021 Alaska Principal of the Year

"Bill Pagaran is a true warrior for the Lord. A man of vision and hope, of prayer and joy. Men like this are rare. You could do no better than to read this book and heed his counsel. A wealth of faith-growing exercises await you!"

Dave Arnold
Executive Producer, Adventures in Odyssey

"It's the passion in how *Rise Above It* is presented that speaks deeply to one's heart. Here, (in these pages) the hope and tools you need can be found to embrace and love the life you live."

Jonathan Maracle
Director, Broken Walls

"Bill Pagaran presents a bold and loving message of hope that prevents suicide in Alaska. Bill and his team love the Indigenous people of Alaska and have dedicated years in service. They love all the people of Alaska and this book will help each individual learn to rise above the challenges in life. I heartily recommend Bill, this book and his teams."

Crystal Collier
President/CEO Seldovia Village Tribe, IRA

"*I commit to life!* This is the most powerful pledge someone can make at any age. Thank you to Bill and the powerful activities outlined in this book for inspiring and teaching tangible ways to make that commitment. As I've traveled to all corners of Alaska and work as a school counselor, I see the tremendous suffering and isolation people feel — we need what this book teaches! I hope this book lands in the hands of as many people as possible so we can save lives, build hope, and commit to life!"

Angelina Klapperich
Miss Alaska 2017, and Alaskan public school counselor

RISE ABOVE IT
HOPE FOR YOUR LIFE'S JOURNEY

By
William Pagaran

PALMER, ALASKA

William Pagaran
1040 W. Beylund Loop
Palmer, AK 99645

Visit our website at *https://www.youcanriseaboveit.org/*

Printed in the United States of America

Rise Above It: Hope For Your Life's Journey/ Pagaran, William

ISBN: 978-173793830-9 Print

ISBN: 978-173793831-6 eBook

LCCN: 2021918330

TABLE of CONTENTS

ABOUT THE AUTHOR

Bill Pagaran, a performer, clinician, educator and mentor, can usually be found somewhere drumming high atop a good-sized mountain. Whether he's in his beloved "hometown" in the Matanuska-Susitna Valley of Alaska or traveling the world, he will always be sharing his inspiring message to "Rise Above It" and emphatically telling everyone he meets, "Don't Let the Rhythm Stop!"

The majority of Bill's time is spent as president of Carry the Cure, Inc. He uses his passion and his natural ability for reaching the unreachable, to drive this non-profit organization. He employs clinical tools and cultural traditions to offer suicide prevention and healthy life-choice skills that bring hope to at-risk Alaskan Natives and other Native Americans.

Bill has a B.Ed. in Secondary Education and keeps his teaching certification current. He is also a certified QPR Suicide Prevention Gatekeeper Instructor. One of Carry the Cure's most active programs, The Committed to Life Program, is a high-energy, multimedia interactive school assembly that gives students reasons to commit to life. Bill believes in raising up a generation that uses their unique gifts and abilities to enrich the lives of those around them, and he is living proof that it is possible to successfully overcome a difficult childhood.

Bill is part Tlingit (Alaskan Native) and part Filipino, and therefore lightheartedly refers to himself as a "Tlingipino." His natural "Native" sense of humor sets those around him at ease from the start, and his understanding of his heritage and culture allow him to speak a language of love and truth to other First Nations peoples, in a way that is graciously received and appreciated by villages and reservations alike.

Bill is also a serious percussionist who has a B.A. in Music. He's been a drummer nearly from birth, maybe because he was often papoosed in his musician father's baby-backpack during gigs. After winning a full-tuition percussion scholarship at the University of Oregon, he went on to perform, tour, and record music professionally. Bill is the author of an instructional percussion book entitled, *Drumming in Half the Time*. Currently, he tours and records with the internationally known Native American band, Broken Walls. The group has earned many indigenous music awards in North America and communicates a message of purpose, hope, and reconciliation through their music. Bill chooses to use his gift of percussion to inspire youth to pursue their dreams and "commit to life."

Although Bill enjoys traveling, his true joy comes from spending precious time with his beloved wife and children.

HOW TO USE THIS BOOK

This book is a Teacher's/Learner's/User's Guide.

That means that it is written to offer everyone hope. Since it is simply a guide, there are many ways to use it to help yourself and others to *rise above it*. Be creative! My desire is that the words, ideas, songs, and activities in this book will inspire overflowing hope. So once you have hope, give it away to others around you. Hope is contagious!

Here are some thoughts and suggestions to help guide you as you use this book:

- Read and be inspired by the personal stories, wisdom, insights, concepts, and truths contained in the book. As has been said, "Truth will set you free."[1] Feeling free from the hurts and pains of the past is a marvelous thing!

- Choose one or more activities from each lesson as they best fit your group, classroom, or event.

- This book is written for all ages; however, some activities (as written) are described more for specific age groups (i.e. elementary, middle school, high school, young adults, etc.). Every lesson can be adjusted to fit any age group, even adults. Just use the basic idea in a section of the lesson and adjust it to your own group's specific age range and group dynamics as needed by using your own wisdom, experiences, insight, knowledge, creativity, and skills.

- Use the activities as supplements to your own lesson or event.

- Use lessons or parts of lessons as a weekly lesson plan in your class or workshop. There is more than enough material in each lesson for you to use in one class setting or session, so if you are planning to use a full lesson for your class, you can divide it up to be used over several days.

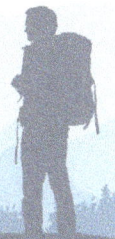

PROLOGUE

My story is not your story, but your story and mine could be alike.

This *Rise Above It* hike was really like the illustrated story of my life.

I know what it's like to be rejected, abandoned, abused and filled with hopelessness. I almost gave up. I was depressed and suicidal at one point of my life. I could've been a negative statistic person. I could've stayed on the low road that would have led to my personal destruction, but I found help. Thanks to answered prayers, people who cared and the wisdom of others, I learned how to rise above the fear, pain, shame, and hurt of my past. I learned how to forgive those who hurt me. I was able to gain victory and freedom over the drugs, alcohol, and other addictions that were destroying my life. I was able to rise above it.

I have an amazing wife, awesome children, and I'm happy. I get to play, perform, and record music around the world. I get to do what I dreamed of doing when I was a boy. If you open your heart today, you can learn how to rise above it all — all that would try to take you down.

If I can rise above it, you can rise above it!

The more I thought about this hiking event and how it related to my life, the more I realized that I was not the only one who has learned to rise above it. I have many friends who have also risen above challenges in their lives. The challenges they once faced may have seemed impossible to overcome at the time, but they did overcome them. Although their stories may be different from mine, my friends learned how to live in victory, freedom, happiness, and fulfillment. Every one of those friends has become a successful person.

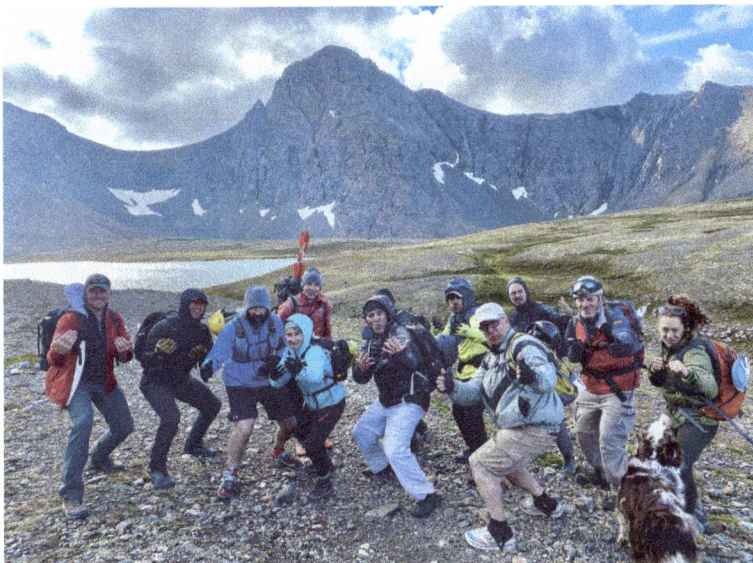

So, I began to invite some of my friends to take this hiking journey with me up South Suicide Peak in order to make a public statement to all people — that we can rise above any challenges in life. I also wanted to make a statement that "together, we are better!" To my delight, I was able to gather a doctor, a nurse, a record-breaking mountain runner, several ultra-marathon runners, two "ninjas" from the *American Ninja Warrior* TV show, a military pilot, veterans, musicians, pastors, a counselor, governmental leaders, youth, a personal fitness trainer, a teacher, and even a grandmother. Once my hiking team, support team, and honored guests were invited and the hiking event date was set, I realized that many more people could benefit from this event if we created a video and a resource guide to accompany it. I began thinking about what I wanted to accomplish through the Rise Above It video and resources. The team and I came up with a list of some of the challenges we have risen above, so that we can teach you how to rise above them, too. That list became this book you hold in your hands.

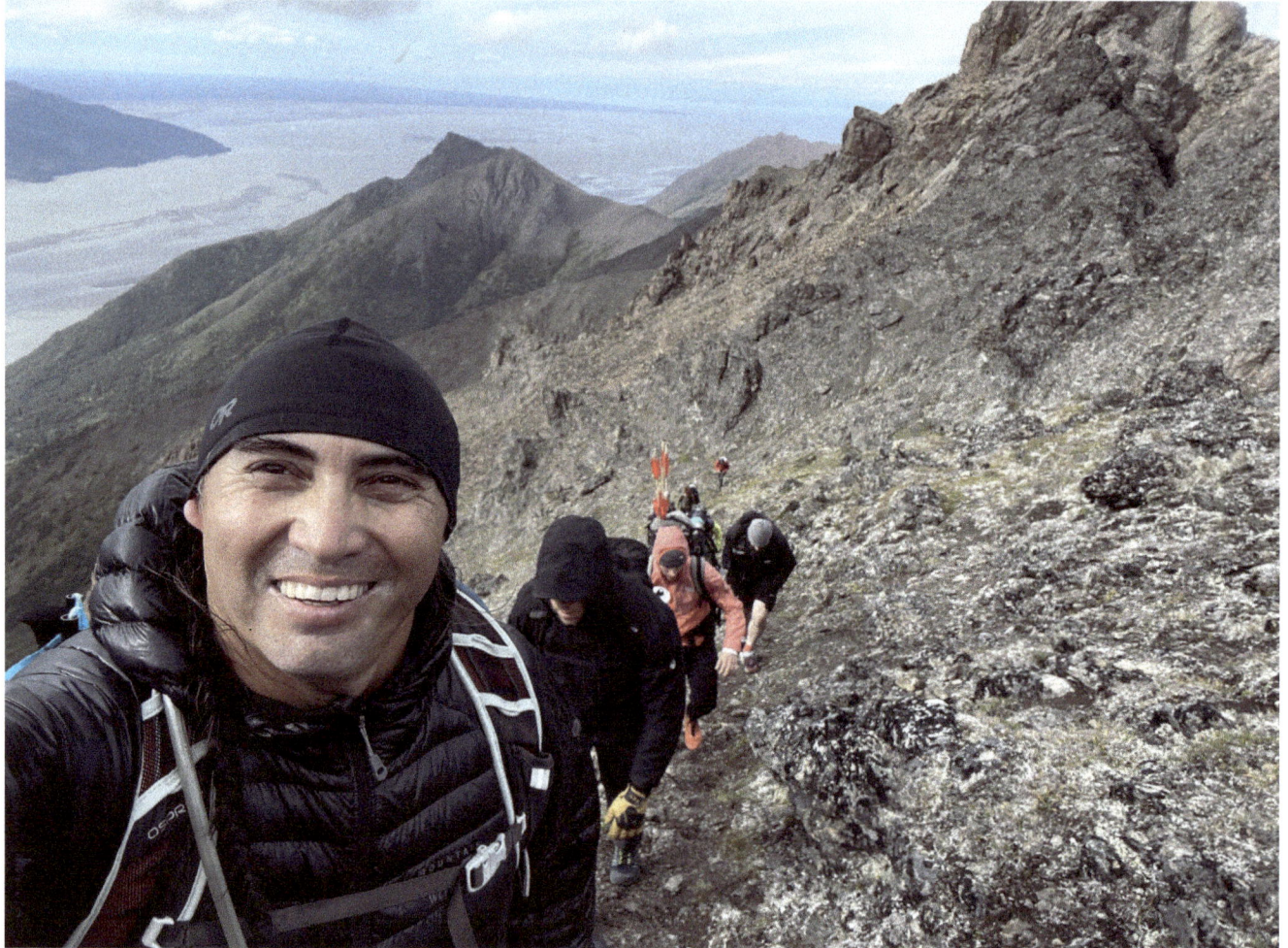

We were not able to address all the challenges of life in this resource guide, but we believe this is a good starting place. This has been, and still is, a cooperative effort from our team.

We all rose above it. Now, we are calling you out as warriors...find strength, learn to forgive, ask for help from your friends. Dream, bounce back, love, serve, give to others, be whole and be what you've been created to be. Do what you've been created to do, and Rise Above It!

If we can rise above it, you can rise above it!

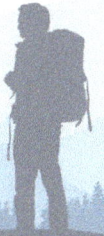

PREPARING FOR THE JOURNEY

Preparing for any good hike, especially in the Alaskan wilderness, you need to have a backpack filled with all the things you need for a safe and enjoyable journey. You'll need a current map, GPS, compass, proper clothing, food, water, emergency supplies and other items to ensure you'll arrive at your destination—and return to the trailhead—in good shape.

Because there are so many dangers and unpredictable things that can happen in the mountains or on the trail, I prefer to take a hiking partner or two with me whenever possible. That way, we can be there for each other if something goes wrong. In addition, I always tell others where I'm going and when they can expect my return. When I hike new trails, I have a GPS map app on my phone that allows me to share my new hiking adventure with my family. Once again, this can be helpful in the event of an emergency. All of which is to say that we need to be prepared for our journey.

Our journey in life is like a hiking adventure. It is filled with beauty that can captive your heart, or a tragedy that can crush it. It's filled with exciting and exhilarating moments, as well as some moments that are intimidating. It's filled with opportunities and options with unknown outcomes. Sometimes in life, I feel like I'm fighting for every step I take. It's a lot like when I'm hiking up a steep ridge: There's great effort and I may be already exhausted. But I know that if I keep moving forward I will be rewarded with an amazing view. I learn and experience something new on every hike I take. Hiking journeys like these are so much like our life.

This Rise Above It Guide is packed full of useful life skills and tools that will help you to face any challenge, climb any mountain and learn to rise above it. My hope is that you will unpack these tools and use them as needed. In addition, I hope that you will help others when you see that they are in need.

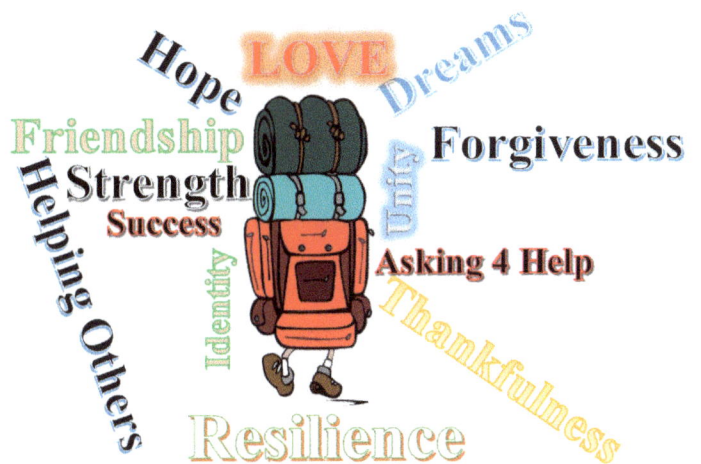

LIGHT UP THE WORLD

SUBJECT:
HOPE

! ATTENTION GETTERS

💬 QUOTES & THOUGHT SHOTS:

A. "Paths to dreams are many. So just hike on a higher one if you get lost."
~ Amanda Pagaran

B. "Looking up reminds me I have much to live for." *~ Amanda Pagaran*

C. "The darker it is, the brighter the twinkle of the stars above you."
~ Amanda Pagaran

D. "Work on having good character; it's a sure gateway to hope." *~ Amanda Pagaran*

👁 VIDEO CLIP:

Hope to Rise Above It[1] ▶ *https://youtu.be/cn7JxtCIQzs*

🗣 DISCUSSION:

1. Read Thought Shot A from above. Have you ever gotten sidetracked from your goal or dream, but ended up with a better one? Tell about it.

2. What do you think Thought Shot C really means? How can dark times in our lives result in some good, or be used for good?

3. Read Thought Shot B. What are some things that "Look up" might mean?

4. What helps you to keep looking up?

5. What have you seen other smart people do to help themselves and others to keep looking up?

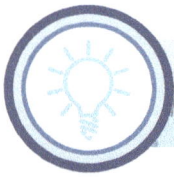

DEFINITION/INSIGHT

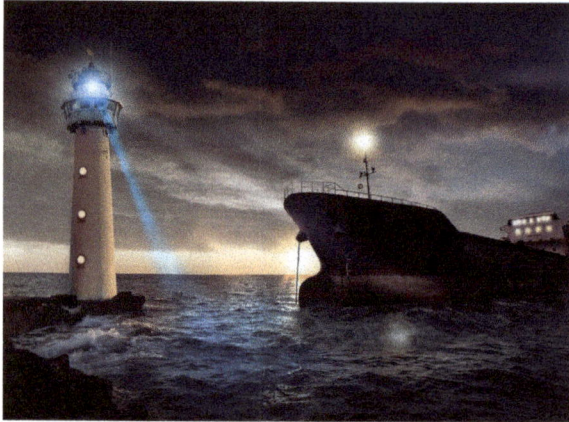

Hope is an anchor to our soul, a light to our path, a reason to live another day, and the fuel that ignites our dreams. The best hope is anchored in love. Hope is a powerful tool against depression, addiction, poverty and racism. Hope helps us to break through the hardest times and situations. Hope can be found in the drum that I play, the song that I sing and the prayers that I dance. Hope helps us to forgive the unforgivable and live the unimaginable. Hope has no racial, social, political, tribal, geographical or religious boundaries. Hope can protect you, help you prosper, and give you a future.

Hope opens your eyes, gives you strength, causes you to soar like an eagle and shine like a star. Hope can "wow" you like the northern lights and stir your compassion for others. Hope can keep you from shame. Hope can save your life. Hope is limitless; it has no end. Hope pours into our hearts through love. Hope has a name and hope has a face. It can show up any place. Hope is found in faith and in people, and all creation exudes it. Hope is like water; we can't live without it.

So, if you have hope, share it with others. Give it away, because you can't outgive hope.

ACTIVITIES

ACTIVITY #1: Commit to Life Vow & Poster

1. Have everyone say the Carry the Cure's Committed to Life Vow out loud, repeating after you, or reading it aloud.

2. Then the group can create a unique Committed to Life poster.

3. Have all the students and teachers who are present, sign it.

4. Get an ink pad and have each student put their thumbprint on the poster. Feel free to create a thumbprint design together. The group could put their thumbprints in a shape to create a heart, school logo, church symbol, or something else that represents your group or community.

5. Have as many people as you can, sign the "Committed to Life" poster that you created (i.e. students, teachers, parents, elders and other community members).

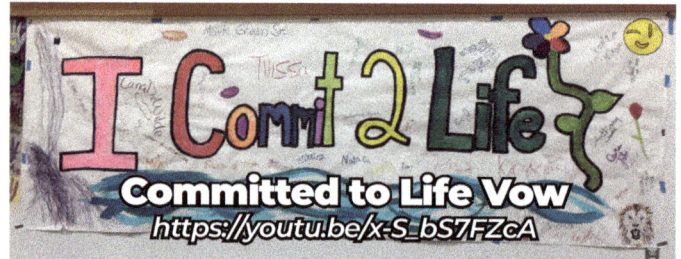

Committed to Life Vow
https://youtu.be/x-S_bS7FZcA

I vow to commit to life and pursue my purpose.
Whether times are good or bad,
whether I have money or not,
even if I'm sick,
when I'm alone or lonely,
I CHOOSE LIFE!
When there's too much pressure,
or when I've lost hope,
I'll ask for help.
I am valuable.
I am loved.
There's a good plan for my life.
I have a purpose.
I COMMIT TO LIFE!

Display your poster in a public area for all to see. Some good places might include the foyer of the school, the gym, or the tribal center.

ACTIVITY #2: Hope Tree

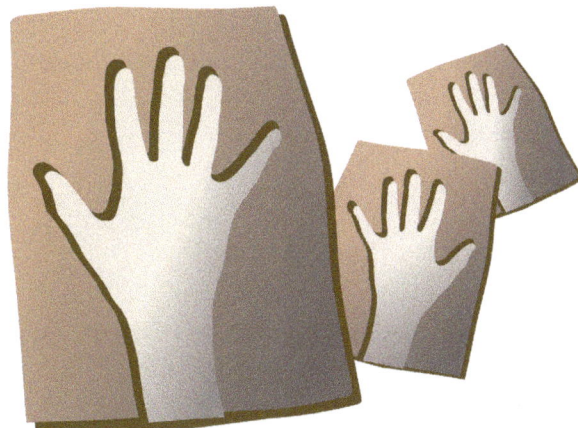

1. On a large poster, have several students trace their hands from the elbow to their fingertips. Make sure each hand is open to help create the branches of the tree.

2. Find some green construction paper and create one or two leaves for each student in your class or group.

3. Give each student five minutes to consider what gives them hope. Have each student write it on their leaf or leaves.

4. Hang the hope leaves on the branches of the hand trees.

5. Consider writing your tribal values or healthy core beliefs as the roots of the tree.

6. Display the poster in a place where all can see.

DISCUSSION:

1. Have students share what they wrote on their paper leaves, and why they wrote it.

2. Ask them how they can help others add "hope leaves" to their Hope Trees.

3. Ask them for other project ideas that might spread hope in their community.

FOLLOW-UP IDEA:

Help grow HOPE in your community! Consider having the students create extra hope leaves and randomly give them out to other students, teachers and community members. This can be more effective if you find someone in your community that you don't know well, someone having a tough day, or maybe an elder that needs a lift to their afternoon. The next class day, have the students share the responses of the people they gave the leaves to.

Consider writing this at the bottom of the leaves they make to give away: "If you need a little extra hope, visit: ⊕ *www.carrythecure.org/resource.html*"[2]

JUST THE FACTS: *SCIENTIFIC FINDINGS*

Hope makes you healthier and happier

"[Researchers] found those with more hope throughout their lives had better overall physical health, better health behaviors, better social support and a longer life. Hope led to fewer chronic health problems, less depression, less anxiety and a lower risk of cancer."[3]

https://hfh.fas.harvard.edu

Hope can help you heal[4]

https://www.cnn.com/2013/04/11/health/
hope-healing-enayati/index.html

Married couples who embrace hope are more likely to stay married for life[5]

https://www.focusonthefamily.com/marriage/
restore-hope-for-your-marriage

Hope saves lives[6]

http://www.qprinstitute.com

Hope helps people live longer[7]

https://www.psychologytoday.com/us/blog/pressure-proof/
201303/5-ways-hope-impacts-health-happiness

Hope helps reduce mental illness[8]

https://pubmed.ncbi.nlm.nih.gov/28953841

Hope can increase academic performance

Hope helps people to achieve their goals in life

Hope increases our productivity in work, school, or play[9]

https://www.scirp.org/pdf/PSYCH_2018032715484959.pdf

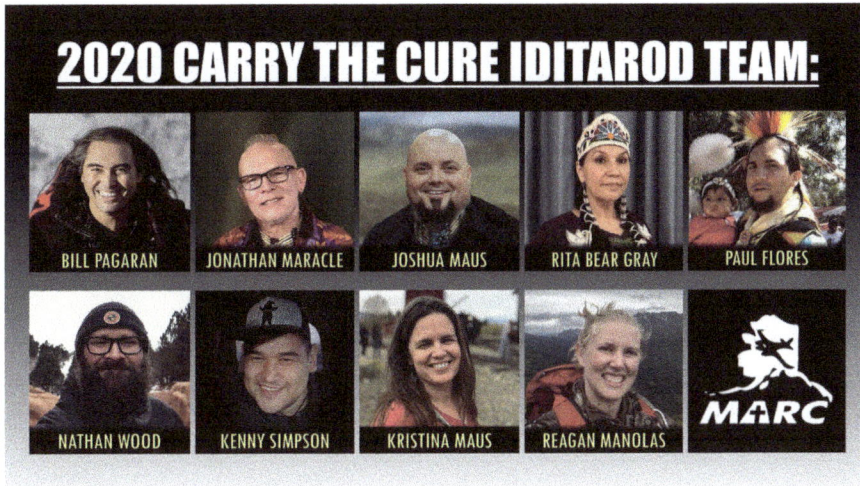

2020 CARRY THE CURE IDITAROD TEAM:

BILL PAGARAN · JONATHAN MARACLE · JOSHUA MAUS · RITA BEAR GRAY · PAUL FLORES

NATHAN WOOD · KENNY SIMPSON · KRISTINA MAUS · REAGAN MANOLAS · MARC

HOPE FROM THE TEAM

Rita Beargray

- "Choose hope to be the anchor in your life."
- "Follow the ancient pathways where the good way is."
- "We will be known forever by the tracks we leave." ~ *Dakota Proverb*

Jonathan Maracle

- "Hope is the one thing we have when all else fails. When it seems there is no hope is when we must cling to hope."

Reagan Manolas

- "Hope is like the stars. The darker the night, the brighter they shine."

Marla Rowland

- "Let hope shape your future."
- "You can rise above any situation and achieve your dreams." ~ *Lailah Gifty Akita*[10]
- "Once you choose hope, anything's possible." ~ *Christopher Reeve*[11]
- "Hope is the joyful and confident anticipation that something good is going to happen [in your life]." ~ *Joyce Meyer*[12]

Amanda Pagaran

- "Where your hope is, power awaits."
- "Base your hope on good, and you will not be disappointed."
- "Hope gives your dreams wings."

Bill Pagaran:

- "Your past pain shouldn't guide your future, let hope show you the way."

Paul Flores

I once gave a graduation speech. I told the graduates that I had a work of art with me that I looked at every day for inspiration. I held up a rectangular wrapped gift for them to see. I told them this work of art gets redone every 20-30 years. Every time, it's remastered with all the best parts of the past rendition. It's one of the oldest pieces of art to ever be created, but even today, when people look upon this work of art, they can't help but feel inspired and hopeful for the future. I held up the gift and told the students that I brought with me the freshest most current rendition, in fact, it was just touched-up just this morning. I told them that as they prepare to take this next step in life, they're going to face trials, excitement, ups and downs. And if they ever feel tired and down, and they need to regain their focus, strength and purpose, just remember this beautiful work of art. Then I tore open the gift and held it up for all of them to see. They looked wide-eyed into a large rectangular mirror. As they peered into their own reflections, I told them that with every generation, by the laws of nature, they're bloodline has grown stronger and better. You have all the best qualities of your parents and grandparents and back through your ancestors. You are a beautiful work of art, the best version of your bloodline to date. There's no other quite like you. You are the masterpiece of generations.

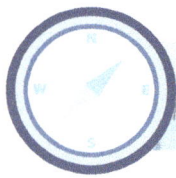

GPS: *WHAT DIRECTION DO I TAKE*

Do you want more hope? Then look for it in others, and if it is a good hope, follow them. Hope is contagious, so when you have found hope, pass it on. Your words are seeds, so if you speak hope, you plant hope in others.

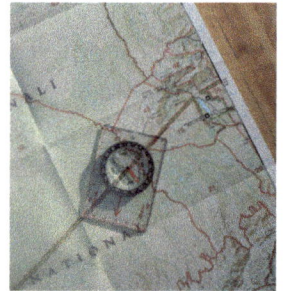

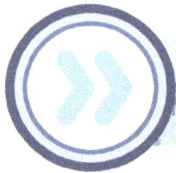

APPLICATION

Share hope with others today. List a few activities/ways to share hope. Here are some that you can use to jump-start your own list:

Serve at a homeless shelter or soup kitchen.

Help an elder by mowing their lawn, taking out their garbage, cleaning their house, cutting some firewood.

Help someone who is disabled or has special needs.

Speak some encouraging words to a friend, peer, family member or even someone in your village.

Write down some of your talents, interests and gift ings in a journal. Write how it makes you feel when you share that talent or gift with others.

Make a list of places you'd like to visit someday.

Write down a short-term goal that's achievable soon, as well as a dream that you can reach for in the future.

14

Here's a really cool list of simple things that anyone can do called, "57 Ways to Spread Kindness and Brighten a Day." Examples: "1. Smile at a stranger; 2. Put change in an expired parking meter; 3. Send someone a handwritten card; 4. Hold a door open for someone; 5. Drop dinner off for an elder."[13]

For more ideas from this resource, visit this link: 🌐 *https://charityideasblog.com/2011/10/26/57-ways-to-spread-kindness*

Journal about, or reflect on, one or more of these questions:

- How do I feel when I am engaging in hope or kindness?
- How can I experience more hope or be kinder toward myself?
- How can I express hope or kindness in interactions with others?

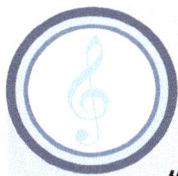

🎼 SONGS TO TAKE YOU HIGHER

I ♥ MUSIC

Listen online or through your favorite music app.

"Trust in You" by Lauren Daigle

"Hope" by Natasha Bedingfield

"Song of Hope (Heaven Come Down)" by Robbie Sheay Band

"Song of Hope" by Avishai Cohen

"Here Comes the Sun" by The Beatles

"Better Days" by One Republic

"I Believe That We Will Win" by Pitbull

"I Dare You" by Kelly Clarkson

"Now is the Time" by Broken Walls

"Fly" by Broken Walls

"Happy" by Pharrell Williams

"Don't Worry, Be Happy" by Bobby McFerrin

"Somewhere Over the Rainbow" by Israel "IZ" Kamakawiwo'ole (originally Judy Garland)

"Walking on Sunshine" by Katrina and the Waves

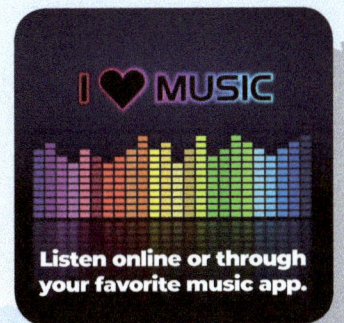

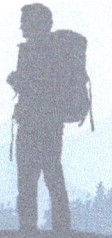

CHECK YOUR TIRES &
KEEP YOUR SEATBELT ON

SUBJECT:
BALANCE IN LIFE

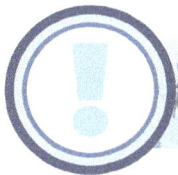

ATTENTION GETTERS

QUOTES & THOUGHT SHOTS:

A. "Life is a journey that must be traveled no matter how bad the roads and accommodations." ~ *Oliver Goldsmith*

B. "Faith gives you an inner strength and a sense of balance and perspective in life." ~ *Gregory Peck*[1]

C. "Life is like riding a bicycle. To keep your balance, you must keep moving." ~ *Albert Einstein*[2]

D. "Balance, peace, and joy are the fruits of a successful life. It starts with recognizing your talents and finding ways to serve others by using them." ~ *Thomas Kinkade*[3]

E. "Seek the good, and your life will fall into balance." ~ *Amanda Pagaran*

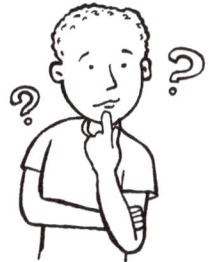

VIDEO CLIP:

Rascal Flatts - Life is a Highway (From "Cars"/Official Video[4] https://youtu.be/5tXh_MfrMe0

DISCUSSION:

1. In the Rascal Flatts' version of this song that you listened to at the beginning of the lesson, it says, "Life is a highway. I want to ride it…" List some of the things you can do to make sure you don't have a breakdown that keeps your "vehicle" from taking you down this exciting highway of life?

2. Pick one of the following quotes from the song, and explain what you think it means:
   a. "When you knock me down, I'm back up again."
   b. "The roads are rough."
   c. "Tell 'em we're survivors."

3. Did any of the quotes at the beginning of this lesson stand out to you? Why? What do you think it means?

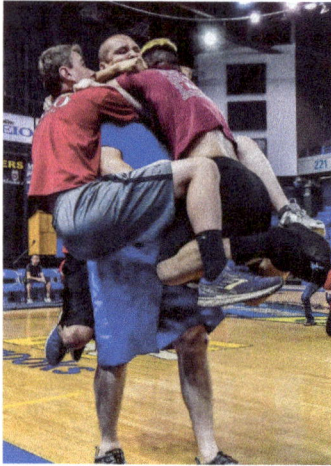

Native Youth Olympics Game: The Four Man Carry[5]

▶ *https://youtu.be/A7sJnuACWi4*

This Alaskan Native sporting event is a good illustration of how a person needs to build strength and skill to balance the four areas of his or her life.

If you decide to have students try it instead of just letting them watch video clips of it, be sure to get parent permission.

Pre-Planned Skit: Flat Tire Skit

This funny skit is a pantomime that can be done with a minimum of preparation. You will need nothing but eight students and a bit of rehearsing beforehand. (They will act out the parts of a car and the driver):

ROLES:

- **Four students as each of the four car tires.** They are to find a way to look like tires on a car (on knees or squatting with head and arms tucked in, to look roundish).

- **One student as the car trunk.** He/she squats or kneels between the two back tires; has arms crossed with elbows extended forward and head down in a manner that can raise up like a trunk opening.

- **One student as the car seat.** On hands and knees, positioned with head facing toward a side of the car, not toward the front or the back of the car.

- **One student as the driver** who is a light-weight person so he/she can gently sit on the back of the person who is the car seat.

- **One student to stand in the background** and make sound effects for everything (i.e. opening the car door, starting the engine, etc.).

THE SKIT:

The driver walks up and gets in his car, starts it and pretends to drive. (The car actually stays in one place, though it's fun if the different parts of the car bounce in unison in time to the engine sound that the Sound Effects person makes.) Then one of the tires goes flat. The driver turns off the car, gets out, opens the trunk, gets a tire pump out, and pumps the tire back up. Then he puts the pump back, gets in the car and drives some more...until...another tire goes flat! This process repeats four times total, each time with a different tire. (It's fun for the actors and the audience if each tire going flat is progressively noisier and more dramatic.) Each time the driver gets more frustrated. Finally, he drives off confident that all the troubles are behind him. Then, all at once, in unison, all four tires blow! Here the driver just drops his head in his arms and loudly (in a funny manner) cries (or whatever funny response seems right to the actors).

DISCUSSION:

1. How is the Four Man Carry game a good illustration of how a person needs to build strength and skill to balance the four areas of his or her life?

2. Did you enjoy the Flat Tire Skit?

3. Have you ever had a day in which everything seemed to go wrong like it did for the main character in the skit? Are there preventative things you can do that may help you avoid having too many of those types of days?

4. Are there ways you can prepare yourself to be able to successfully get through those types of days when they do come? How can you help others when one of their bad days come?

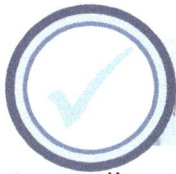

✓ JUST THE FACTS: RESEARCH

According to Dr. Walt Larimore, a nationally recognized family physician educator, best-selling author of 32 books, and award-winning medical journalist, our overall health or wellness has four distinct areas: "Physical, Emotional, Relational and Spiritual." It is vital that each of these areas is in balance with the rest, and that they are working together in order for our lives to move forward in a good way.

I like to relate this concept as a customized four-wheel-drive vehicle. Each tire represents one of the four areas of our wellness. If one tire is low, the vehicle doesn't travel well. If one tire is flat, or nonfunctional, then we can't move forward at all.

Therefore, we must keep these four areas of our life in balance:[6]

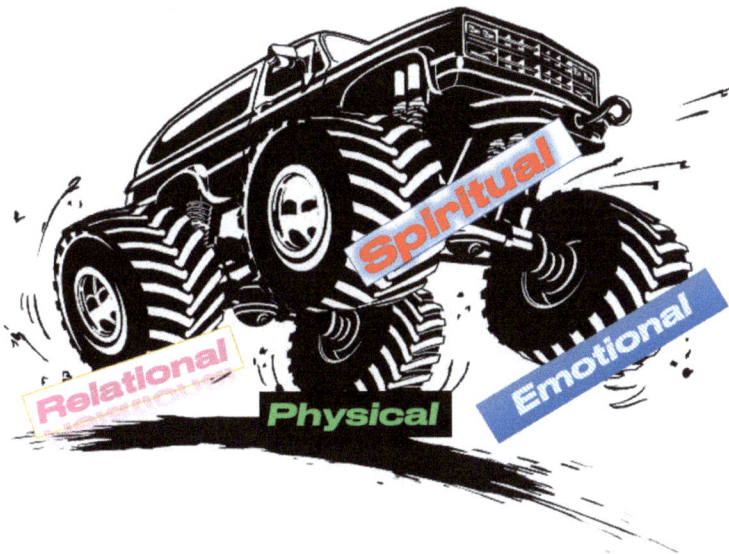

Spiritual
1. Prayer 2. Fellowship 3. Meditation
4. Faith Sharing

Emotional
1. Stimulation/Learning 2. Hostility
3. Stress/Depression 4. Work

Relational
1. Parents/Children 2. Extended Family/Friends
3. Social Support 4. Spouse

Physical
1. Exercise 2. Substance Abuse/Safety
3. Nutritional/BMI 4. Rest

Once you know where you are in each area, you can make the adjustments and get your life in balance.

THOUGHTS FROM THE TEAM

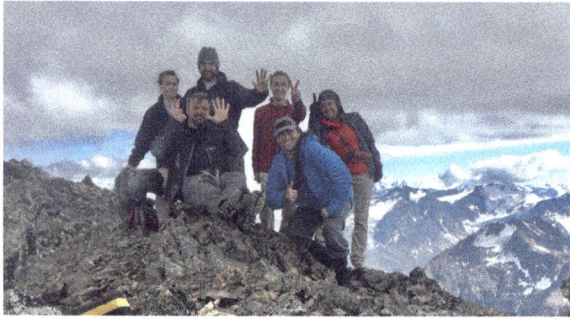

Some people think life is a 40-yard dash; others consider it a marathon. Whatever way you choose to look at it, it's important to run the race to win. If we are going to win in life, we must prepare and protect every facet of our life so that we can make it to the end. Not only that, but we want to enjoy every part of the race we are running.

A common quote is, "It's not how you begin the race, but how you finish." I want to finish life well. To do that, I must consider the four main areas of my life (spiritual, emotional, relational, and physical), and do things that will help me keep strong in each of these areas. Here are a few things that I personally do to keep a strong and balanced life:

SPIRITUAL

I go on prayer hikes, read the Bible, consider how the word of God applies to my life and daily living, listen to lots of worship music, go to church and share the Good News with others.

EMOTIONAL

I practice new music, take classes, work with others, work in the yard or on my home, volunteer, enjoy the outdoors, go fishing and play marimba or drums. These things seem to help keep me from the extreme roller-coaster of life.

RELATIONAL

I spend lots of time with my kids. I love them! So, we have some great meals together, play games, go fishing, talk, do projects together, and more. I've been married a long time to my beautiful wife, Amanda. We go on lots of dates, walk together, talk together, travel together, go to church together, deal with tough situations as a team and serve our community together. I also have many friends who help me stay strong. Relationships are key to running our race in life well.

PHYSICAL

I avoid drugs, alcohol and other harmful substances. I try to eat right. I go on tons of hikes, play some sports, work hard, fish hard and play with my dog. I maintain pretty good sleep habits, too.

I'm far from perfect. I do have weaknesses; however, if I'm mindful of these four things in my life and I attempt to keep them in check, my imaginary four-wheel-drive vehicle doesn't break down as much. We all have seasons in our life when things are tough. I've found that when I go through a tough time, it's often because I've neglected one of these four main areas in my life. I love the illustration of these four areas (spiritual, emotional, relational, and physical) represented by the tires of a customized vehicle. If we keep air in those tires, the vehicle can go almost anywhere.

Remember, in this analogy you are a like a customized vehicle. Your tires, wheels, rims and accessories are different from mine. How you address these four main areas of life will be different from mine. The important thing is that you keep them in balance.

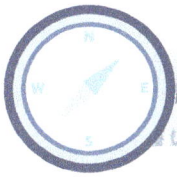

GPS: *WHAT DIRECTION DO I TAKE*

Check your tires! Take an inventory of what you're doing in the four main areas of your life. Make a list of some things you can do to strengthen your weaker areas. If you are doing well in some areas...keep on truckin'!

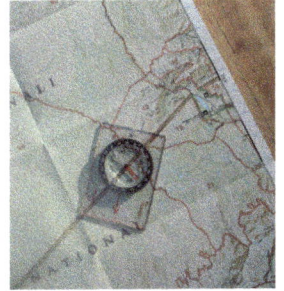

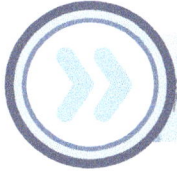

APPLICATION

Most of us have different tastes in music. We have songs to help us to grow in our faith, to lift us when we are down, to build up our emotions, to learn to become a better friend, to appreciate our friends, and to grow stronger.

Divide into groups of four. Each group should find their own songs for the main four areas of life: spiritual, emotional, relational and physical. Each group should try to come up with at least two songs in each area. (If a group finishes early, they can start working on writing their own song!) Once the groups have completed their group tasks, have each member share one of their group's song choices with the entire group, and discuss why they chose it.

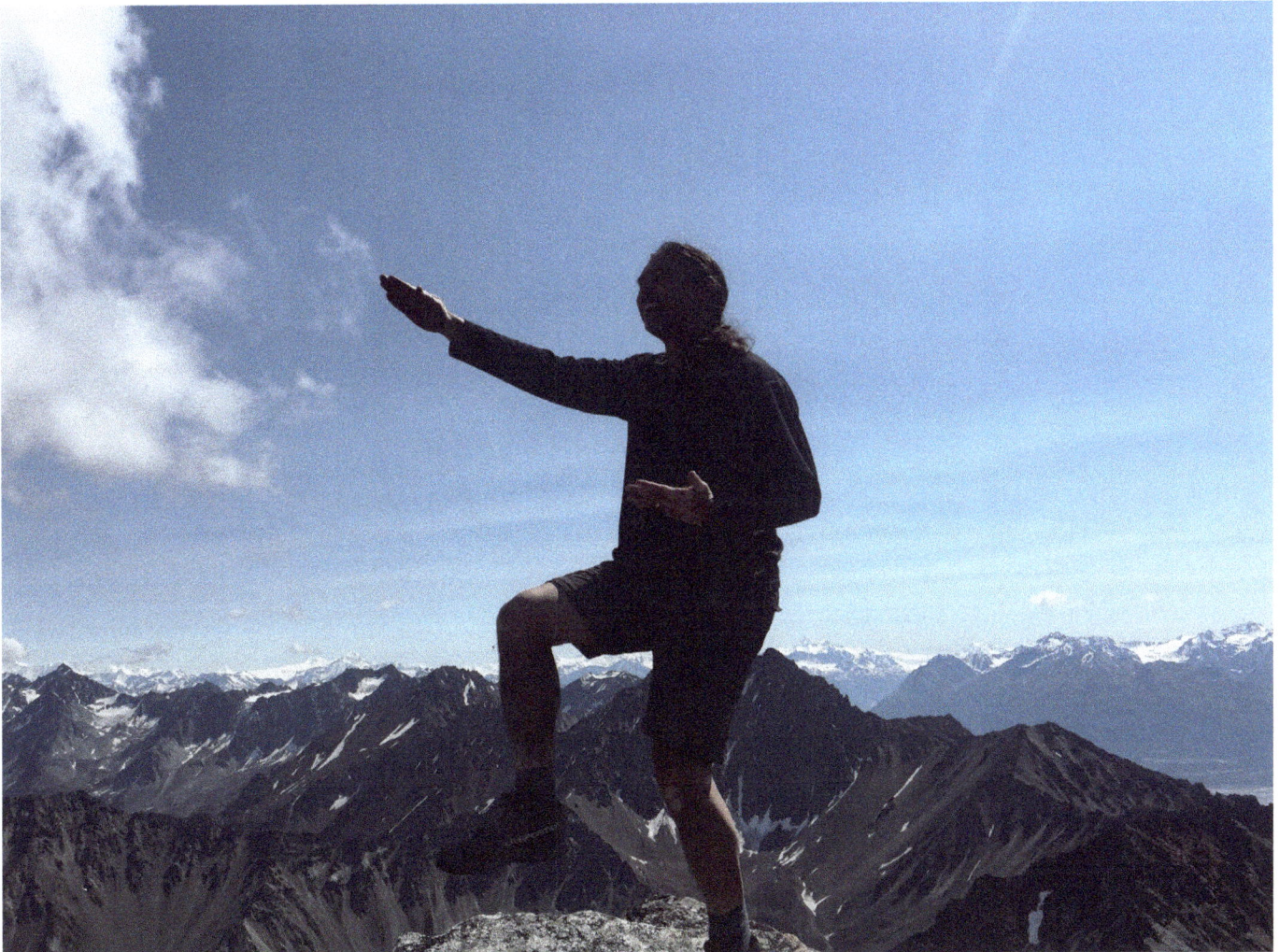

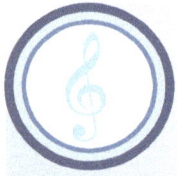

SONGS TO TAKE YOU HIGHER

"Life is a Highway" by Rascal Flatts

I ♥ MUSIC

Listen online or through your favorite music app.

SPIRITUAL
"I Love the Way You Hold Me" by Jamie Grace and Toby Mac
"My Best Friend" by Hillsong Kids *(ALSO RELATIONAL)*

EMOTIONAL
"You Say" by Lauren Daigle
"Headphones" by Britt Nicole

RELATIONAL
"You Raise Me Up" by Josh Groban
"Friends" by Meghan Trainor

PHYSICAL
"Eye of the Tiger" by Survivor

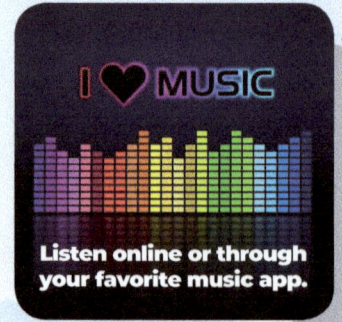

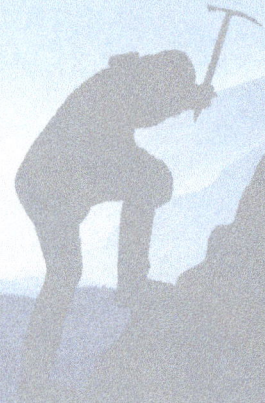

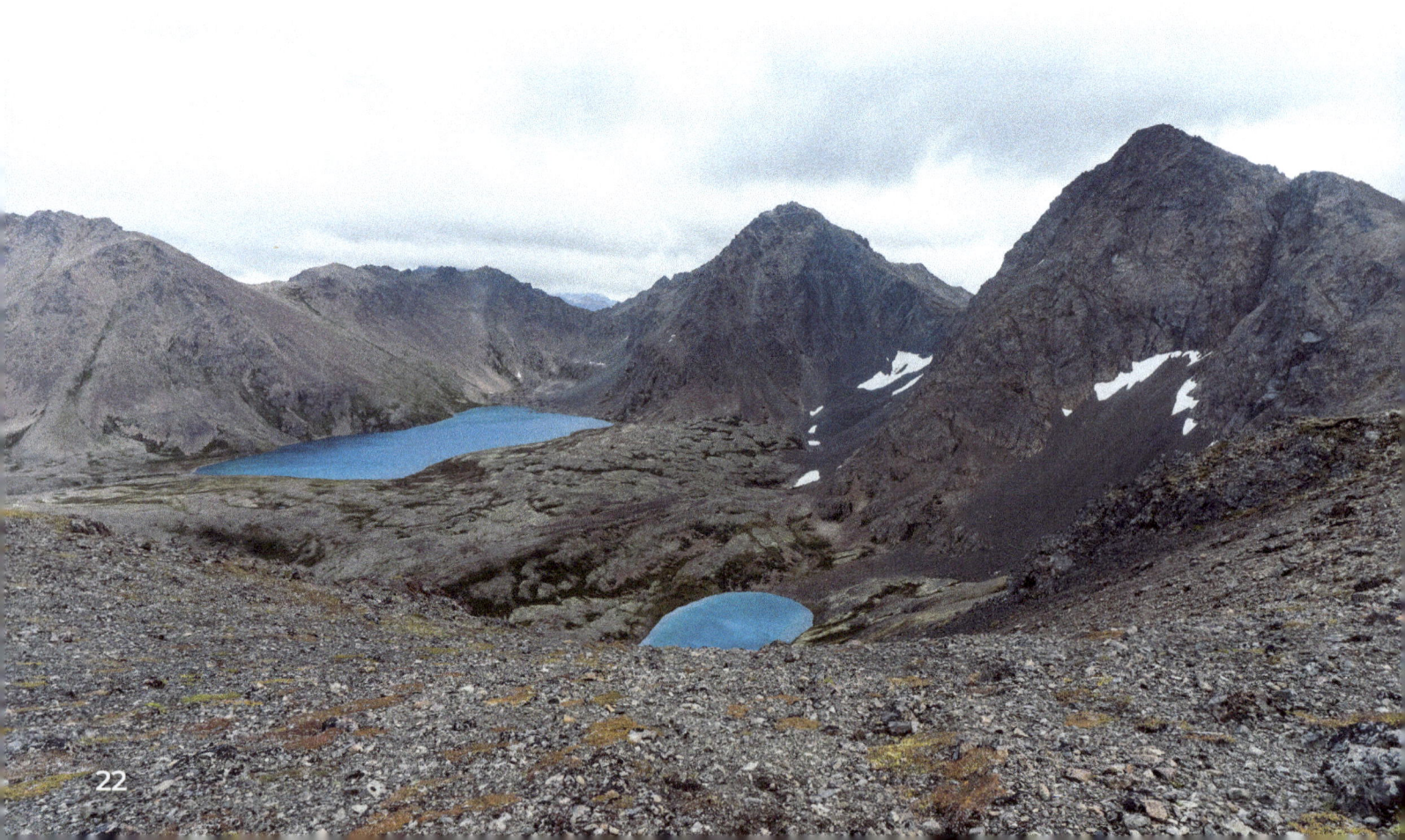

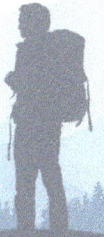

THE NAME GAME

SUBJECT:
KNOWING MY TRUE IDENTITY

Written by Marla Rowland (Carry the Cure, Inc. Team Member)

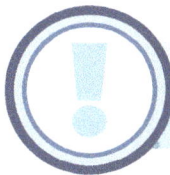 ## ATTENTION GETTERS

💬 QUOTES & THOUGHT SHOTS:

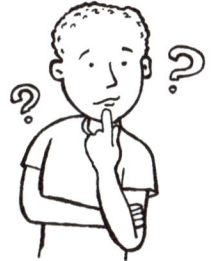

A. "Let go of who you think you are supposed to be and be who you are." ~ *Brene Brown*[1]

B. "Owning your story is the bravest thing you will ever do. When you own your story, you can write a brave new ending." ~ *Brene Brown*[1]

C. "My story matters because I matter. I am absolutely enough." ~ *Brene Brown*[2]

D. "Don't try to change yourself to fit in with bad company...Leave!" ~ *Amanda Pagaran*

E. "Care about others, be considerate and compassionate, but don't become a "people pleaser". "People pleasers" have trouble finding out who they truly are, and have trouble becoming who they were meant to become." ~ *Amanda Pagaran*

F. F. "Always be a first-rate version of yourself, instead of second-rate version or somebody else." ~ *Judy Garland*[3]

👁 VIDEO CLIP:

Rocky Balboa Motivational Inspirational Speech To Son 1080p YouTube 720p[4]

▶ *https://youtu.be/N8h8LsaktnQ?t=60*   or   ⊙ *START: 1:00:40 END 1:04:53*

Scene: *Robert Balboa, Jr. barges into the restaurant to have a serious talk with his father, Rocky. He demands that they speak outside. Robert begins to give his Dad a piece of his mind. He expects to confront his father about who he truly is, but finds his father's love and understanding is deeper than he imagined.*

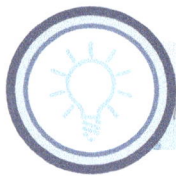

DEFINITION/INSIGHT

IDENTITY:

Learning the truth about ourselves, and coming to honor and celebrate our uniqueness, is an important choice we can make. There is a wholehearted life we can choose to live when we let go of who we think we're supposed to be and embrace who we are.

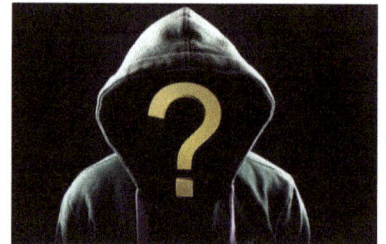

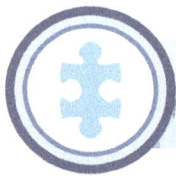

ACTIVITIES

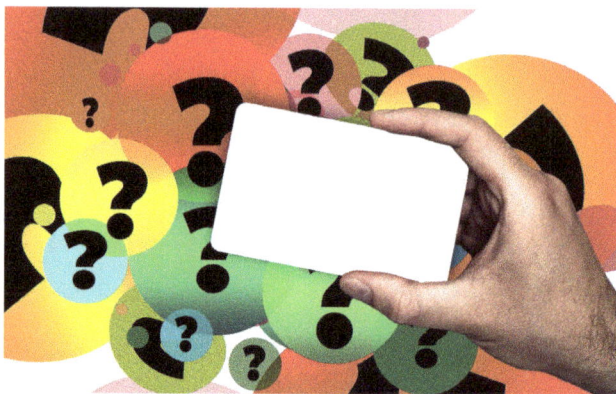

Activity #1: The Name Game

This can be played with any number of people. Divide into two teams (teams can be anywhere from 3-30 people).

On strips of blank paper, instruct every person to **write the name of a famous or well-known person** (from history, sports, government leaders, etc.; can be living or dead). Have them fold the paper in half and place in a bowl or bag.

First Round: Taking turns as teams, one person from each team picks a name out of the bowl. His teammates then try to guess whose name is on the paper by asking questions that he/she can only answer by saying "Yes" or "No." Time each team. The fastest one wins.

Second Round: Do the same thing, only this time the one who has picked the name has to use charades only. No talking or sounds. Just body movement. Time each team. The fastest team wins.

Activity #2: What Does My Name Mean?

If you have access to the internet, do a search for the meaning of your first name. Here is a good site[5]: 🌐 *https://www.sheknows.com/baby-names*

Write down the meaning of your first name.

Get into groups of 3 to 4. Taking turns, each person will share what their name means and how they responded to what they found. Did it resonate with them? Encourage them? As each person shares, the others in the group are encouraged to identify the positive qualities they see in that person, affirming them by speaking it out. (This is an important step in learning to do this for each other. To build up rather than tear down.)

Activity #3: NAME ACROSTIC

This is an art project—art is therapeutic!. If preferred, it can be done as a stand-alone activity separate from the lesson time.

Provide quality colored paper, markers, pens, stickers, magazines, etc. Each person should write the letters of their first name across the top or left-hand side of their papers. For each letter of their first name, they will choose and write down one positive adjective that begins with each letter of their first name. (You can search online for "adjectives beginning with the letter "A", etc. to help you).

EXAMPLES

Karen		**Gabe**	
K	Kind	**G**	Giving
A	Artistic	**A**	Athletic
R	Reliable	**B**	Bubbly
E	Enthusiastic	**E**	Easy-Going
N	Nice		

This is a great exercise to help each person identify the good qualities within themselves. Encourage them to take this paper home and hang it on their bedroom wall or somewhere they will see it often, to help them begin to believe the good things that are true about who they are.

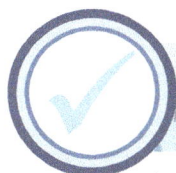

JUST THE FACTS: *STATISTICS*

"A person's name is the greatest connection to their own identity and individuality. Some might say it is the most important word in the world to that person. It is the one way we can easily get someone's attention. It is a sign of courtesy and a way of recognizing them."[6] ~ *Joyce E.A. Russell*

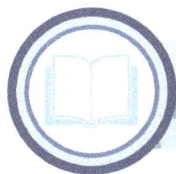

LESSON

♫ SONG:

Lauren Daigle - You Say (Official Music Video)[7]
▶ *https://youtu.be/slaT8Jl2zpl* *Lyrics available in description.*

DISCUSSION:

1. How many of you can relate to the lyrics?

2. Have you ever felt like you weren't enough? Have you felt like you don't measure up?

3. What types of things can help when you feel like that?

As we grow up and experience life, people sometimes speak hurtful words to us or about us. Words that are painful, words that make us feel we're not worthy, or maybe not wanted. In those places of pain, we can begin to believe lies about ourselves. We doubt our value, our importance.

These harmful words can feel like 'labels' that people put on us. And those 'labels' can feel like truth, they can become our identity. It's how we see ourselves. Labels like unwanted. Loser. Stupid. Worthless.

Circumstances in life can keep us from knowing the truth of who we really are...until our minds are filled with lies that cause us to isolate, fight, run away, freeze, or numb ourselves to stop the pain.

We need to stop believing what others say we are and start asking "Who do I say I am?"

🗣 PERSONAL STORY: Nick Hanson

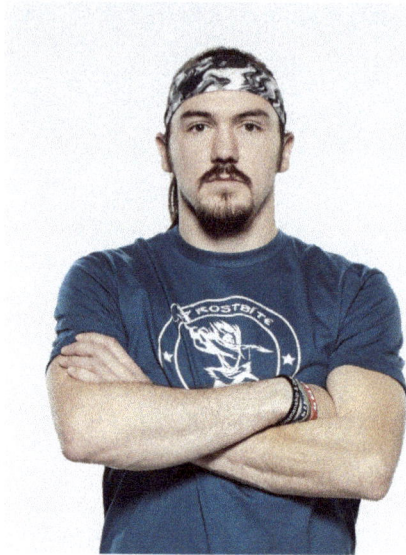

Check out Nick's stories here:

🌐 *https://www.instagram.com/tv/ B6ZaZJ8FIRg*

AND

🌐 *https://www.anchoragepress. com/sports_and_outdoors/ nick-hanson-s-long-journey-to- american-ninja-warrior-and-his- passion-for-promoting-community/ article_c906ae88-7e89-11ea-850e- 7b14ccccd9cd.html*

AND

▶ *https://youtu.be/vAqLUAOT7Lw?t=85*
(additional clip at 5:06)

Tell the whole story of Nick Hanson, from depressed, suicidal teen in the village—to becoming the Eskimo Ninja Warrior who now uses his platform to spread a message of LIFE and HOPE.

APPLICATION:

We must break agreement with these lies about ourselves. Just like Nick did. We must take the 'labels' off . Only then can we discover the truth of who we really are. We are not what people say we are. We are not what we've done in our past. We are not what people have done to us in our past. We are all created with unique personalities, giftings, and destinies.

The good news is that lives which were driven by anxiety, fear, shame and guilt can be replaced by lives driven by love, courage, compassion and connection.

📢 DECLARATIONS:

These are some of the declarations that help us understand that we have choices and that we can come to believe the truth about who we are and gain confidence in our identity. (Leader: choose the ones you want to share and have students repeat these after you.)

- I am unique and special. There is no one else like me.
- I am worthy of love and belonging.
- I am enough.
- I am not a victim. I take responsibility for my life and choices.
- I have confidence in myself. I have a voice.
- I can say what I want and what I need.
- I was created for a purpose.
- I am free to be me.
- I can let go of unhealthy relationships.
- I connect with healthy supportive friends.

- I accept myself as imperfect but as lovable and acceptable.
- I am able to deal with my feelings (feeling them and letting the negative ones go).
- I view mistakes as learning opportunities. It's ok to make mistakes.
- I can think, make good decisions, solve problems and figure things out

SONG:

Katy Perry - Roar (Official)[8] ▶ *https://youtu.be/CevxZvSJLk8   Lyrics available in description.*

APPLICATION

When you begin to know and walk in your true identity and what you were born to do, you begin to ROAR! And when you do, it impacts and influences others around you. You were born to change the world. It doesn't have to look like Nick. It's whatever you were made to do. Believe in yourself; believe in the gifts you have. Take advantage of the opportunities you've been given and watch as more doors open before you!

Personal Follow-Up Activities and Ideas:

- Spend some time journaling
- Write your own poem or story
- Take a hike and think on it
- Share your thoughts with others
- Write a song.

- Create a drama, illustration or game
- Make your own video
- Start a positive group or club
- Create a related art project
- Or do something inspired just by you!

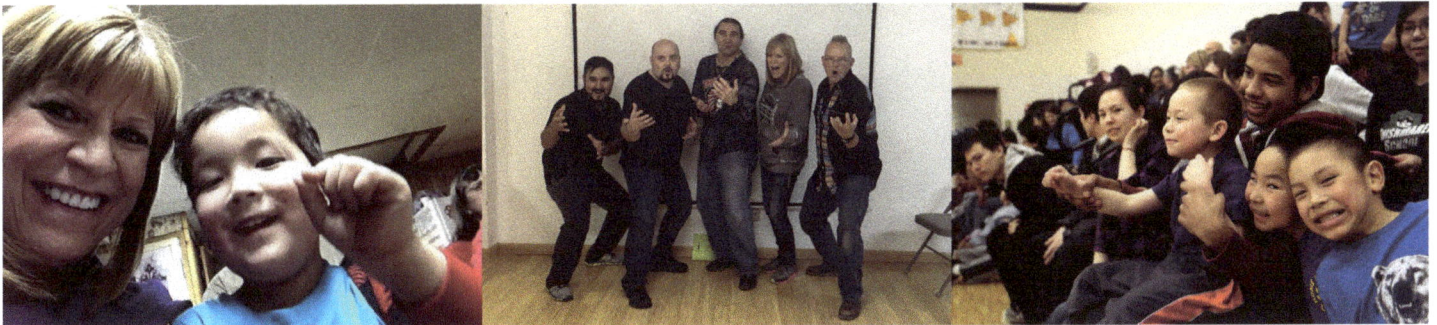

SONGS TO TAKE YOU HIGHER

"You Say" by Lauren Daigle
"Roar" by Katy Perry

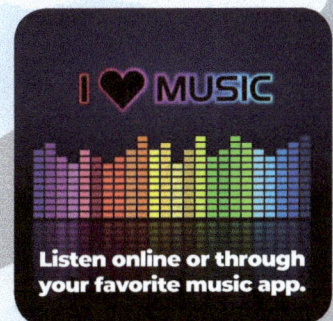

I ♥ MUSIC

Listen online or through your favorite music app.

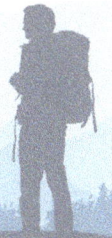

REACH FOR THE HEAVENS

SUBJECT:
DREAM BIG, DREAM OFTEN, HOPE ALWAYS

Written by Denali Tshibaka (Yuyanq' Ch'ex Team Member)

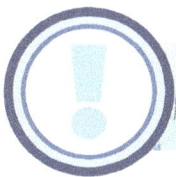

⚠ ATTENTION GETTERS

💬 QUOTES & THOUGHT SHOTS:

A. "I am not afraid to dream. You first have to start with a dream. Build your castles in the air and give it foundation. Without a dream, you are not going to get anywhere." ~ *Kofi Anan*[1]

B. "There are some people who live in a dream world, and there are some who face reality; and then there are those who turn one into the other." ~ *Douglas H. Everett*[2]

C. "Nothing is impossible; you just have to know who to ask." ~ *Amanda Pagaran*

D. "Dream big and dream often; dreamers are the ones who start the landslides that accomplish the impossible." ~ *Amanda Pagaran*

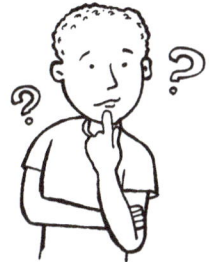

👁 VIDEO CLIPS:

Prince Ntwali's Dream[3] ▶ *https://youtu.be/6PQUt1RRZeg*

Martin Luther King Jr's 'I Have A Dream' Speech[4] ▶ *https://youtu.be/gdTpU5WZHHM*

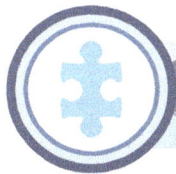

🧩 ACTIVITIES

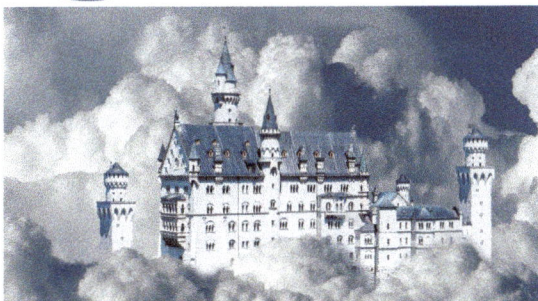

GAME: Castles in the Air

Materials: *Construction paper; scissors; pencils, pens, markers, colored pencils, or crayons*

Messy Rating: *Minimal*

Duration: *30 to 45 minutes*

Cost: *Classroom supplies (+$4.00 for construction paper)*

This exercise is designed to help participants build their own castles in the air by writing or illustrating their dreams and sharing them with others. Through this simple but significant act of putting their dreams to paper and sharing them with others, participants give their dreams — their castles in the air — a foundation. They are taking the first step toward actualizing their dreams and living out their hopes.

Ask each participant to take a piece of construction paper and, using a pair of scissors, cut it into the shape of a cloud. Encourage them to have fun with the size and shape of the cloud they create. After all, just like clouds, dreams are unique. Next, ask the participants to write down or illustrate one of their dreams. Challenge them to be creative. For instance, if they are writing down a dream, they could express it in a poem or song. If they wish to illustrate a dream, they might consider using symbolism and culturally significant images to depict it.

Instruct the participants that their dreams can be about anything. For example, they can be:

- Dreams about their family, village, or tribe;
- Dreams about a character trait they would like to develop in themselves;
- Dreams about what they want for their future;
- Dreams about a skill they want to master or an obstacle they want to overcome
- Dreams about a change they want to see in the world around them.

Give the participants 20 to 30 minutes for this exercise. When they finish, give them another 10 to 15 minutes to share their dream with at least one or two other people.

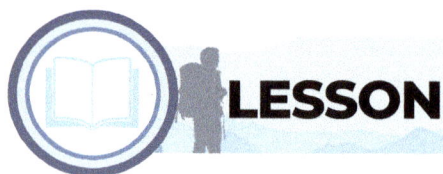

LESSON

The simple act of putting your dream to paper is the first step toward fulfilling it. It is the first stone in the foundation for your castle in the air and the first taste of the hope your dream holds.

Advice/lesson (What do others say that have learned to rise above?):

All humans are dreamers by nature. Every achievement and every hope fulfilled begins with a dream. Dreams determine the destinies of individuals, communities, tribes, nations, and generations. Our dreams challenge us to scale mountains and inspire us to reach for the heavens. They guide us, embolden us, and define us. Dreams give us hope and determine our futures.

This world needs you — it needs your dreams and your hopes. You matter. Your hopes matter. Your dreams matter — they have the potential not only to change your life for the better, but also to change your community, your world, and even the course of history. Martin Luther King Jr.'s successful leadership of the civil rights movement began with a dream that gave hope to millions of black and white Americans. The suffragette movement began with Susan B. Anthony and Elizabeth Cady Stanton's dream that women would be given the right to vote. Their shared dream gave hope to millions of women across the country and resulted in the Nineteenth Amendment, which guaranteed women the right to vote.

Your dreams hold incredible power, which means you hold incredible power. You do not have to be rich, famous, or talented to make your dreams come true or help others. So dream often, dream boldly, and dream of forging paths others would fear to tread. In the words of the great poet, Edgar Allen Poe, dream "dreams no mortal ever dared to dream before." Pursue your dreams large and small with passion and perseverance. As you do, you will experience hope along the way, a hope you can share with a world that desperately needs it. Build your castles in the air, then give them foundation!

🗣 PERSONAL STORY: Denali Tshibaka

I am only 16 years old, so most of my hopes and dreams have not had enough time to come to fruition. There are, however, some that have begun to blossom. In fourth grade, I discovered that I had a knack for writing — specifically, for writing poems. I would write about nature, holidays, spiritual matters, and anything else that weighed on my mind and heart. Over the years, I began to develop a dream for my poems — that they would, one day, make an impact on others, whether large or small.

So, I wrote whenever I felt inspired. Whether the topic was uplifting, depressing, goofy, or reflective, I did not care. I soon combined my poems into one large compilation. I spent years adding one poem at a time to my growing collection. *One day,* I continued saying to myself, *one day, I will have the ability to share these with the world. One day, someone somewhere will feel impacted by my words.*

Fast forward seven years to August 29th, 2020. I was honored to participate in the Rise Above It hike. Before we began, several people were asked to say a few words. I presented a poem I had written several years before that relayed my own experience with someone I knew who committed suicide. In that moment, I knew that my dream had begun to come true. My poem was shared with people who could spread it and impact others.

Dreams take some time to come true; most are not instantaneous. Build a strong foundation for your castles in the air, then continue to add to it. My deepest wish for you is that your dreams will one day come true.

HEROES WHO LEARNED TO BE RESILIENT

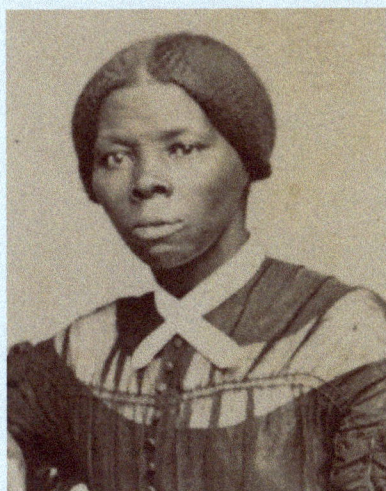

Harriet Tubman was born as an enslaved person in Maryland, but she had a dream to be free. In 1849, Harriet escaped and fled to the North, achieving her dream of freedom. When she experienced the treasure that freedom is, however, she had a new dream — to lead others to freedom. Ultimately, she became one of the most famous leaders of what was known as the "Underground Railroad". Tubman risked her life to lead hundreds of slaves to freedom, including her own family members. In 2016, in honor of her work, the U.S. Treasury Department announced the possibility that Harriet Tubman would replace former President Andrew Jackson, who was a slaveholder, on the new $20 bill. Harriet Tubman was a dreamer whose unshakeable hope and dedication to her dreams changed the world.

DISCUSSION:

1. What did you feel as you listened to Prince Ntwali and Martin Luther King Jr. share their dreams?
2. Do you think it is worth pursuing dreams that might not come true? Why or why not?
3. What do you think the most important part of a dream is?
4. What scares or discourages you most about pursuing your dreams?
5. What did you learn about yourself in doing the Castles in the Air game?

JUST THE FACTS: *STATISTICS*

Research has found that hope is critical to successfully pursuing our dreams. Individuals who are hope-filled are physically healthier and less vulnerable to disease. They have better self-esteem, a deeper sense of meaning, and healthier relationships. They also perform better academically and athletically, and have purpose in life[5]:

🌐 *https://www.mindwise.org/blog/community/the-power-and-science-of-hope*

GPS: *WHAT DIRECTION DO I TAKE*

If you want to become effective at pursuing dreams:

1. Believe in yourself and in your dreams.
2. Do not be afraid to share your dreams with others. They can help, support, and encourage you as you pursue those dreams.
3. Make it a regular practice to have a small dream each week that you can pursue and achieve by the end of the week.
4. Read stories about other dreamers and learn from their failures and successes. Draw inspiration from their examples.
5. Keep a dream journal in which you write down your dreams (big ones and small ones), and how you plan to pursue them.

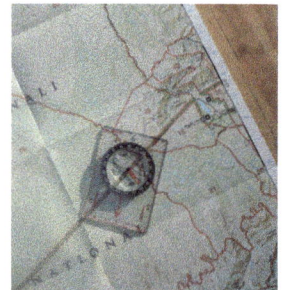

APPLICATION

Work with your classmates to develop a shared dream for your community that you can all pursue together. Once you agree on your shared dream, develop a plan for how you will achieve it. Then work together as a team of dreamers to fulfill your collective dream. Build your castle in the air, then give it a foundation together!

Personal Follow-Up Activities and Ideas:

- Spend some time journaling
- Write your own poem or story
- Take a hike and think on it
- Share your thoughts with others
- Write a song.

- Create a drama, illustration or game
- Make your own video
- Start a positive group or club
- Create a related art project
- Or do something inspired just by you!

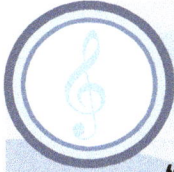

SONGS TO TAKE YOU HIGHER

"When You Believe" by Whitney Houston & Mariah Carey

"The Climb" by Miley Cyrus

"Can't Take That Away" by Mariah Carey

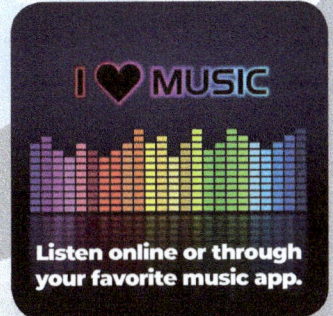

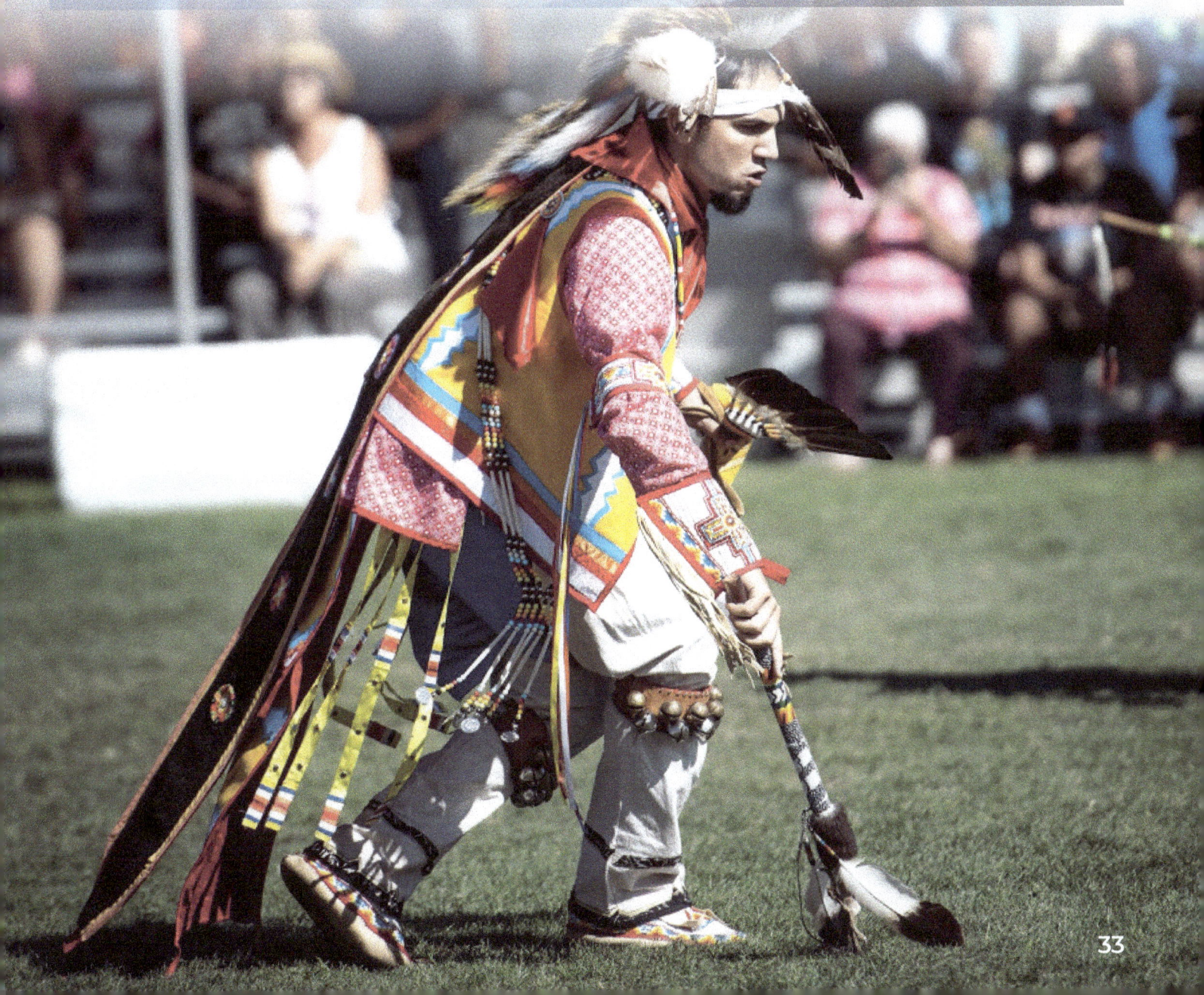

I ♥ MUSIC

Listen online or through your favorite music app.

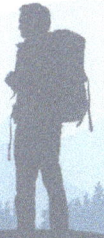

THE STRENGTH OF A GOOD FRIEND

SUBJECT:
FRIENDSHIP

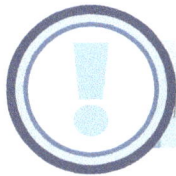

ATTENTION GETTERS

QUOTES & THOUGHT SHOTS:

A. "Show me your friends and I'll show you your future." ~ *Anonymous*

B. "You can make more friends in two months by becoming interested in other people than you can in two years by trying to get other people interested in you." ~ *Dale Carnegie*

C. "If you go looking for a friend, you're going to find they're very scarce. If you go out to be a friend, you'll find them everywhere." ~ *Zig Ziglar*

D. "Friends are those rare people who ask how we are and then wait to hear the answer." ~ *Ed Cunningham*

E. "A good friend can tell you what is the matter with you in a minute. He may not seem such a good friend after telling." ~ *Arthur Brisbane*

F. "Good friends don't keep deadly secrets." ~ *Anonymous*

G. "If you make friends with yourself you will never be alone." ~ *Maxwell Maltz*

H. "Build a bridge, not a wall, and you will find a friend...at the other end." ~ *Anonymous*

I. "The royal road to a man's heart is to talk to him about the things he treasures most." ~ *Dale Carnegie*

J. "Be a giver of kind words, the one who refreshes the thirsty and dry. Who needs more sand when they are standing in a desert!" ~ *Amanda Pagaran*

K. "A good friend shines truth and hope into our lives, like a light in the darkness. Be that light and a friend will always be on the horizon." ~ *Amanda Pagaran*

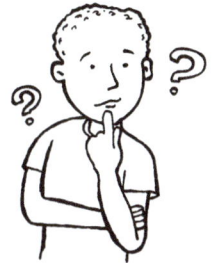

VIDEO CLIPS:

Will Smith - Friend Like Me (from Aladdin) (Official Video) https://youtu.be/1at7kKzBYxI

Caminandes 3: Llamigos https://youtu.be/SkVqJ1SGeL0

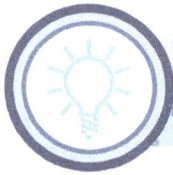

DEFINITION/INSIGHT

Developing good friends is the best way to avoid bullying.

Finding what we have in common is what brings friends together, but learning how to grow through our diff erences is what keeps us together.

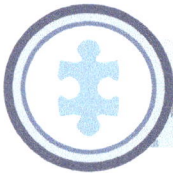

ACTIVITIES

ACTIVITY #1: "That's Me!"

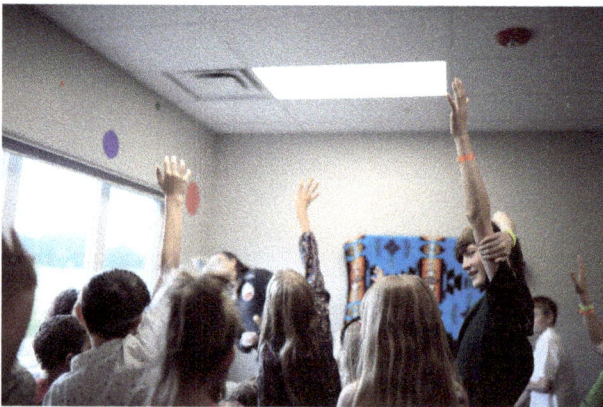

One person stands in front of the group and shares a fact about themselves, like their favorite color or favorite animal. Everyone who also shares that favorite thing stands up and yells, "That's me!"

Kids love this game because it's interactive. They get to share their favorite things, there's fun in not knowing what each child is going to say, and there's yelling.

It's a win all around.

DISCUSSION:

1. What are some of the things most of us have in common?
2. Were you relieved to find out that you weren't alone?
3. Does knowing you have something in common with someone make you more likely to be friends with them? Why?
4. All people need to be loved, listened to and affirmed. Do you agree with that statement? Why or why not?
5. How does knowing you have something in common with others make you want to help them when they are in need?

ACTIVITY #2: "Friendship Chain"

Each child is given a slip of construction paper. On their paper, they write what they think is the most important quality in a friend. Those slips then get taped together to form a chain, which can be hung in the classroom and referred to throughout the year.

DISCUSSION:

It's important to see what we have in common, but it's also important to value our differences. Does seeing this friendship chain help you to get a better picture of how our differences can be linked together to form a stronger friendship?

1. Do the qualities we feel are most important help to bind the other qualities together?

2. An old, wise saying goes, "one can be overpowered; two can defend themselves; but a strand (chain) of three cannot be quickly broken." Do you agree that there is strength in numbers? Why?

3. Describe some situations in which it would be important to link/stick together.

4. How will you connect with others around you?

ACTIVITY #3: "In Common"

This game is a great activity for breaking down barriers. Kids are put in small groups, ideally with a mix of kids they aren't already friends with. Each group then has to find seven (or whatever number you want) things that they all have in common.

The kids learn a lot about each other, but also find out that they have more in common with students from different social groups than they thought.

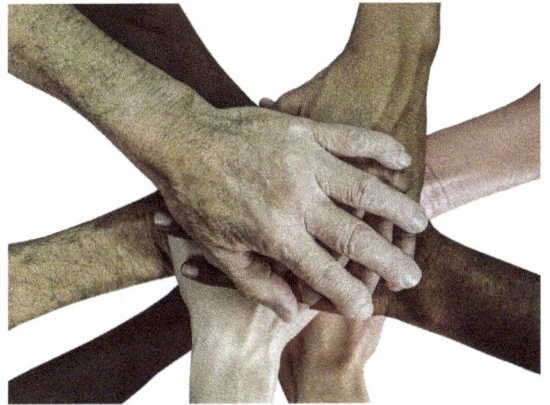

DISCUSSION:

1. After the activity, have a member from each group share what the group has in common.

2. Have students reflect on their thoughts about their discoveries and about what they learned and felt during the activity.

The games above are primarily derived from the following source:

🌐 *https://www.healthline.com/health/parenting/friendship-activities#Middle-School-Friendship-Activities*

Meredith Bland also supplies a wonderful array of communication games for various ages and has some wise insights about the importance of friendship activities, especially for the middle school age group.

"In middle school, friendship becomes more complicated and more important. Between mean girls, peer pressure, and hormones, there's a lot for kids to deal with at this stage.

Friends become more important, typically replacing family members as confidants. Kids develop some of their first deep, intimate friends. They also struggle to be accepted and must learn how to deal with social hierarchies and cliques.

Friendship activities for middle schoolers tend to focus on teamwork and breaking down barriers between kids. They're also a great way to work on how to handle peer pressure and how to treat other people." ~ *Meredith Bland*

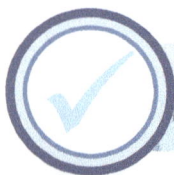

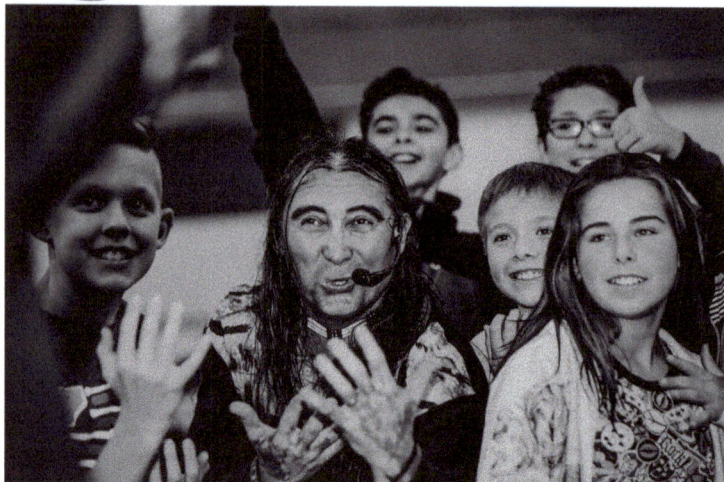

- "Bullying is never, ever the fault of the person on the receiving end of it." ~ *DitchTheLabel.org*
  https://www.ditchthelabel.org/21-facts-about-bullying

- "Finally, [some of] those who bully are more likely to feel like their friendships and family relationships aren't very secure. In order to keep friendships, they might be pressured by their peers to behave in a certain way. They are more likely to feel like those who are closest to them make them do things that they don't feel comfortable doing and aren't very supportive or loving." ~ *DitchTheLabel.org*
  https://www.ditchthelabel.org/why-do-people-bully

- "Friendships are crucial when it comes to bullying prevention. Bullies often target kids who are socially isolated. Kids who have a strong circle of friends are less likely to become victims of bullying." ~ *VeryWellFamily.com*
  https://www.verywellfamily.com/7-characteristics-of-a-bullyproof-friendship-460644

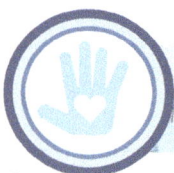

THOUGHTS FROM THE TEAM: *CYBER FRIENDS*

Social media can be a great tool to keep in touch with friends, family and groups that share common interests. I continually use social media to bring encouragement or a ray of hope to others, especially my friends. However, I have on occasion shot off a message to a friend that I wish I hadn't. It usually happens when I'm tired or in a big hurry, and so I didn't think about how the other person might respond to my thoughts. There have also been occasions when Siri, Alexa, or auto text interprets something for me in a bad way and I forgot to proof it before sending it. Whatever the case may be, these kinds of things can cause tension in relationships. It's never my intention to hurt someone with my words, so I try to make it a habit to proofread my messages carefully before sharing them.

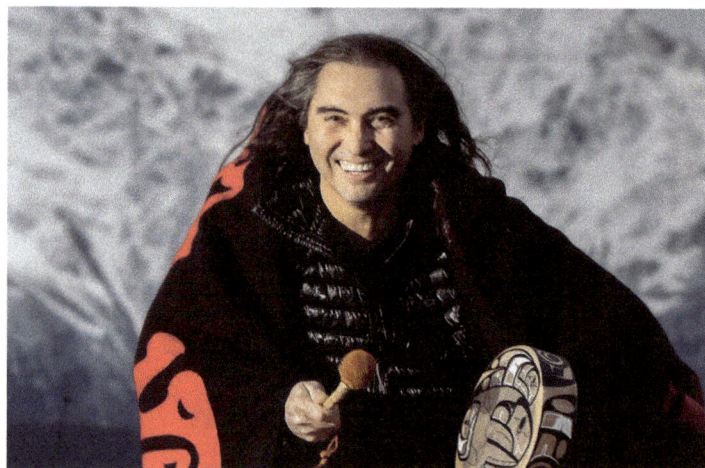

Some people deliberately use social media as a means to hurt others. This is known as cyber-bullying. This behavior is harmful to others as well as to the bullies themselves; potentially leading victims to throughts of worthlessness, helplessness, and suicide. To prevent this type of tragedy, please consider others (and the impact on your own future) before you Snapchat, TikTok, Instagram, Tweet, Facebook, text, send emails, etc.

Before the technology age, we used to say; "think before you speak," or "look before you leap." Now, we must also remember to think before you text. If not, we may find ourselves trying to remove our foot from our mouth or falling into places we'll have a hard time getting out of.

One of the positive things I've found personally about social media is that I'm able to develop friendships with people I've met in my travels throughout the world. Together, we've been able to share our lives' joys, successes and woes. I love receiving encouragement, prayers, fun emojis and virtual high fives from those friends. It's very cool that because we have kept our interactions positive with each other online, it's like a party when we get to see each other again in person.

My hope is that you can develop cyber friends and use your social media in positive ways. It can help turn a bad day into the best one you've ever had. It can help pull you through a difficult moment. It could even save your life. What a delight technology can be when it's used properly.

GPS: *WHAT DIRECTION DO I TAKE*

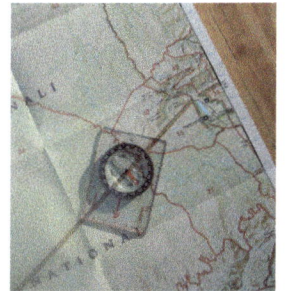

Make some new friends today. Smile at people. Say "Hi," "What's up," "You look great today," or "You're awesome!" Be kind, considerate and compassionate. Share a good (clean) joke with someone. Go to youth groups, sporting events, Native Youth Olympics, games, concerts, church, beading group, chess club, science club. Fish with others, hunt with others, join a sport or go to other school or community events with others. Cheer on the team with them or give them a "high five" after a score. You might also be able to join in with others with some comments about the game or activity. After a few exchanges introduce yourself, and before you know it, you've just made a friend.

Help others you don't know: Open a door, help someone carry their groceries or walk an elder across the street. If you see someone in need, offer to assist them. As the saying goes, "Many hands make light work." Friends value help in a time of need; and helping others often leads to friendship.

When you see someone feeling down, share a word of encouragement. Console them or simply say something kind.

When you are texting someone, stop and consider talking to them in person or on the phone instead of texting. Research proves that it's better for our emotions and better for building good relationships when we are face-to-face or at least voice-to-voice.

Make time and figure out ways to hang around the friends you do have. Learn how to be there for each other in every situation: the good, the bad and the ugly. Encourage, build up, and stand up for each other.

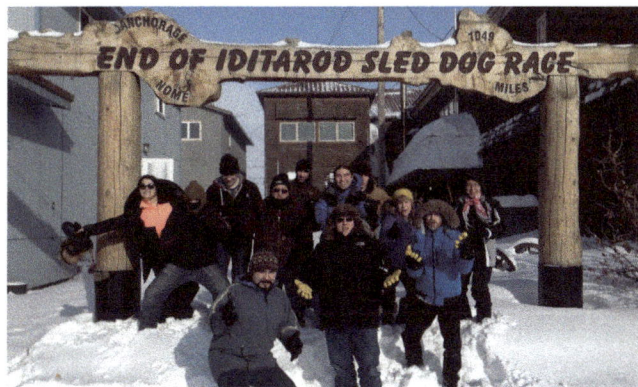

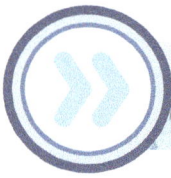

▶▶ APPLICATION

Personal Follow-Up Activities and Ideas:

- Invite people you know to go on a hike
- Have a game night or movie night
- Watch a sporting event
- Go to a youth group
- Find a service project in your community (feeding the homeless, etc.) to volunteer with together
- Start a drum group or a dance group.

You can be the one to start something worthwhile; that's something there's no age limit for.

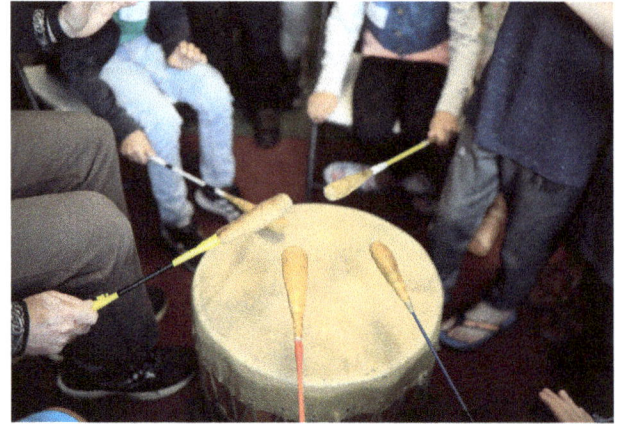

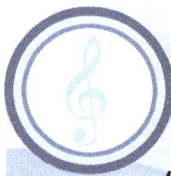

♪ SONGS TO TAKE YOU HIGHER

"Count on Me" by Bruno Mars

"Lean On Me" by DC Talk (originally by Bill Withers)

"You've Got a Friend In Me" by Randy Newman

"The Gift of a Friend" by Demi Lovato

"Find Out Who Your Friends Are" by Tracy Lawrence

"I'll Be There" by The Jackson 5

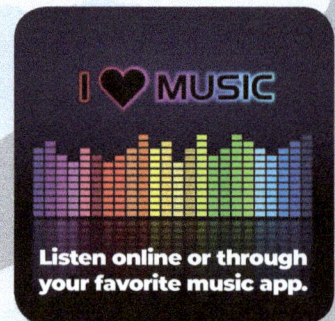

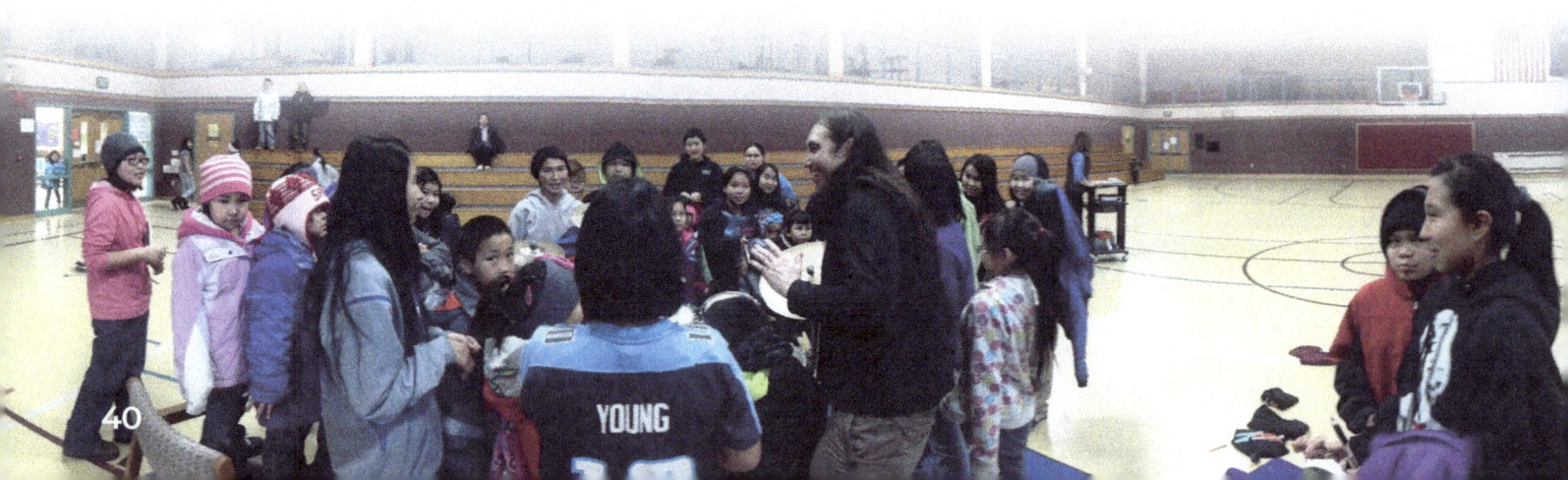

I ♥ MUSIC

Listen online or through your favorite music app.

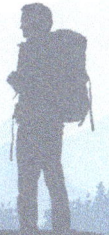

FREEDOM IN FORGIVENESS

SUBJECT:
FORGIVING

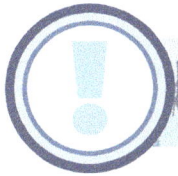

! ATTENTION GETTERS

💬 QUOTES & THOUGHT SHOTS:

A. "To forgive is to set a prisoner free and discover that prisoner was you." ~ *Lewis B. Smedes*[1]

B. "Unforgiveness is like drinking poison yourself and waiting for the other person to die." ~ *Marianne Williamson*[2]

C. "*Forgiveness* and *Trust* are two very different things. It makes perfect sense to FORGIVE. That doesn't mean you have to TRUST that person again, however; why fall into the same hole twice!" ~ *Amanda Pagaran*

D. "The act of forgiving is choosing the high road, the better way. It is the way of the great ones, and it always leads to a good place." ~ *Amanda Pagaran*

E. "A nail in my tire creates a slow leak; if I don't deal with it, I'm eventually going to end up with a flat tire. I think unforgiveness is a slow leak in our soul, in our spirit. When we have a hard time forgiving someone, it really doesn't hurt that person. It ultimately causes the greatest damage to us." ~ *Mark Batterson*[3]

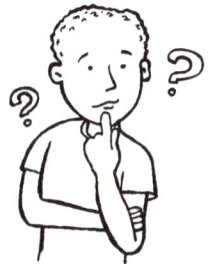

DISCUSSION: *THE QUOTES*

1. What images does Smedes' quote bring to your mind?
2. Does the quote make you want to be a prisoner locked up in a jail, or freed from prison?
3. What kind of freedoms in your life do you long for?
4. What kind of freedoms do you wish for others to walk in?
5. What do you think the Marianne Williamson quote means?

👁 VIDEO CLIP:

The Princess Bride (5/12) Movie CLIP - The Battle of Wits (1987) HD ▶ *https://youtu.be/rMz7JBRbmNo*

DISCUSSION: *VIDEO CLIP*

1. What did you learn about poison from The Princess Bride movie clip?
2. How could that clip relate to unforgiveness?
3. Did you know that in the movie, they both end up drinking the poison? What's the antidote (the cure) for the poison in the movie?
4. Why wouldn't that antidote work if applied to unforgiveness?
5. What antidote do you think might work in real life for curing the poison of unforgiveness?

DEFINITION/INSIGHT

FORGIVENESS:

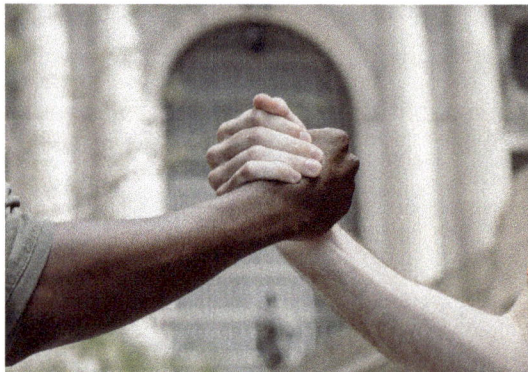

DEFINITION #1:

Forgiveness is the intentional and voluntary process by which a victim undergoes a change in feelings and attitude regarding an offense and overcomes negative emotions such as resentment and vengeance.

DEFINITION #2:

Letting go of your anger at someone.

ACTIVITIES

GAME: Spew

Materials: *Alka-Seltzer, Sprite or 7-Up*

Messy Rating: *Need a towel or two*

Duration: *5 to 20 minutes*

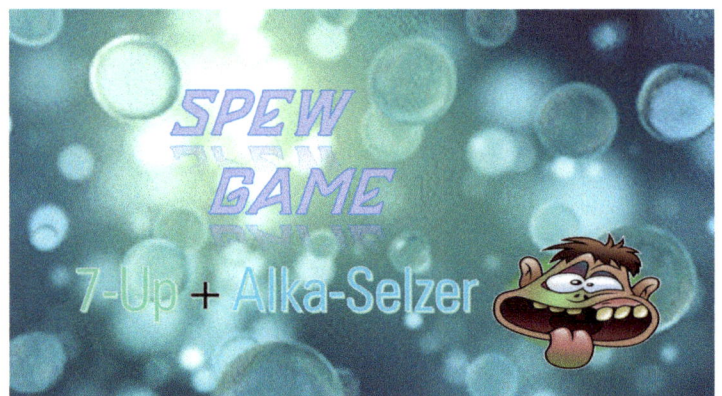

This game/lesson goes perfectly with this lesson on "unforgiveness". Get some Alka-Seltzer and some carbonated, clear drink (e.g. Sprite, 7Up, Ginger Ale, or Squirt). Tell each of your participants to place a single Alka-Seltzer underneath their tongue, but not to swallow it. Don't worry: they won't be able to swallow the tablet with it under the tongue.

Now, give them each a small cup (only about 3 or 4 ounces) of the clear carbonated drink. The object is to see who can hold it in their mouth the longest, but trust me, it will EXPLODE and SPEW out of their mouths! I wouldn't advise swallowing it. It won't hurt them, but *yuck*. They must have at least a couple ounces in order for it to work, but bear in mind that it is not about how much they can drink. It's about how long they can hold it. Have fun!

The Alka-Seltzer tablet represents the offense in our heart. The carbonated drink symbolizes other issues in our lives that stir up our anger, hurt, and/or resentment. When people offend us, it puts pressure in our lives. Then, when they or others "push the right buttons", our hurt and anger build up. If we don't get rid of the offense (i.e., the Alka-Seltzer) in our lives, then we will spew our hurt and anger onto others even if they had nothing to do with the original offense.

The Lesson: If we learn to release the pressure in our lives by forgiving others, we will feel freedom.

DISCUSSION: *THE GAME*

1. What did you learn from the Spew game?
2. How could you relate what happened in the game to any unforgiveness you may be holding in?
3. In the game, what did you learn about other issues in our lives?
4. How do we release the pressure to avoid hurting others around us?
5. What's the antidote (the cure)? How could you counteract the poison?

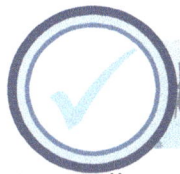

JUST THE FACTS: *STATISTICS*

According to John Hopkins Medicine, unforgiveness can lead to nervousness, fear, worry, high blood pressure, sleepiness, anger issues and a bunch of other medical issues.[5] Learn the benefits of forgiveness: your life depends on it:

https://www.hopkinsmedicine.org/health/wellness-and-prevention/forgiveness-your-health-depends-on-it

LESSON

What Do Others Who Have Learned to Rise Above It Say?

Every person in this world desires to be free. Free to enjoy life and all the good things it has to offer. Free to laugh, sing, smile, dance, hunt, fish, trap, learn, speak our heart, bead, sew, create things and share those good things with others. Free to be ourselves. It feels good to be free! When we walk in freedom others can't take us down by their harsh opinions, criticisms or judgment. When we are truly free, our past doesn't even entangle us. Freedom is a beautiful thing. But, freedom is never free. It comes with a price. Like the men and women in the military who have sacrificed so that we can become and remain a free nation, we must learn how to fight for our personal freedoms on the battleground of life. Otherwise, we can end up holding ourselves as prisoners. A quote by Lewis B. Smedes states this well: "To forgive is to set a prisoner free and discover that prisoner was you."[1] Forgiving others is a great way to set others free of their offense, but it is also vital for us to keep our own freedom in our own hearts and minds.

You might ask yourself, *How can I forgive if I can't forget?*

It is when other people wrong us or offend us that we often lose our own personal freedom and joy.

If you are hurt, abused, lied to, betrayed, abandoned, or rejected by someone — they should apologize, right? If they take or break your stuff, or if they use something without asking — that is wrong, isn't it? When someone hurts you like that, you feel that they owe you an apology. Some people carry that offense in their heart like an IOU. Whenever they see that person who has wronged them, they think in their heart that if the offender doesn't apologize, they will make them pay in other ways. This is what we do sometimes. We don't look at them, we don't talk to them, we don't Tweet, Snapchat, Instagram, Facebook, DM, or email them. We ignore them and run from them to avoid talking to them. Sometimes, we'll go out of our way to avoid seeing them. If we do these things instead of forgiving them, that offense has turned into unforgiveness in our heart, and it hurts us.

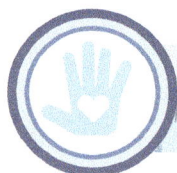

THOUGHTS FROM THE TEAM:

Bill Pagaran's Personal Experience

I learned that holding unforgiveness in my heart towards others only made me feel bad. Often times, the other person didn't even know that they hurt me. They didn't feel my hurt, nor did they feel bad.

Without knowing it, I would hold on to that offense in my heart. The offense inside my heart turned to pain, anger and resentment. If I didn't release that offense, it just got worse, and that in turn made me feel even worse. It could even lead to my own death!

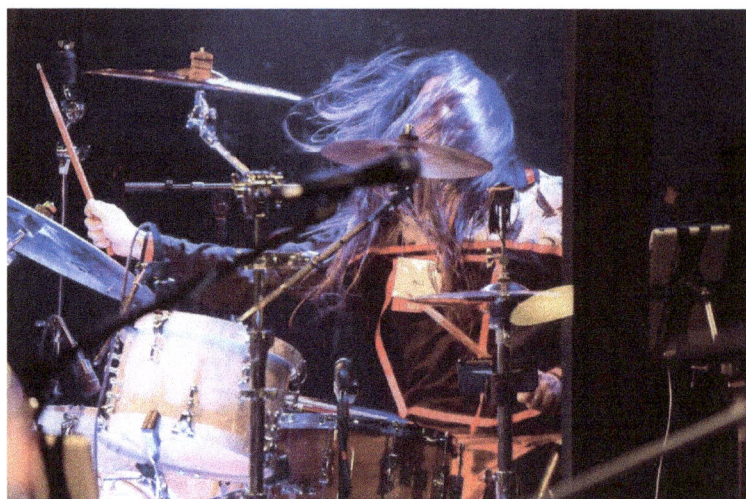

What I really wanted was for them to feel my pain, to suffer and ask me to forgive them, or to pay for what they did to me. Instead, I learned that I was the one who needed to extend forgiveness. As I forgave them and released them from what I thought they owed me, I became free of the pain, anger, and resentment. As I forgave, the power that the offense/hurt had on me was broken off. Not only was it broken off me, but freely forgiving others and tearing up the IOU often (though not always) inspired them to ask for forgiveness from me and others, too.

At first, I thought harboring those hurtful feelings gave me power over them. Later, I discovered that forgiving others of their offense gave me freedom from the hurt, pain, and anger that had held me captive.

You were created for freedom. You were created for joy! Your willingness to release forgiveness can end the war in your personal life, as well as in the lives of those you love.

Remember, the key is forgiving without expecting the other person to ask for forgiveness. This can be really tough. It also might require some extra help from a trusted person. Choose to forgive. Choose freedom. Learn to forgive and forget and experience the true freedom you were born to walk in.

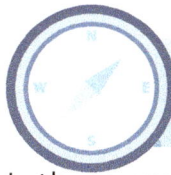

GPS: *WHAT DIRECTION DO I TAKE*

Is there anyone you need to forgive?

1. Talk to your mom, dad, grand-parent, or trusted elder and ask them to help you forgive. This will help you to apply what was shared in the *Rise Above It* video. We need to learn to forgive, live, and give. Learning to forgive leads to living in freedom. When we forgive, we also give the gift of freedom to the person who offended us.

2. Other people you can talk to include your school counselor, teacher, pastor, priest, or youth worker. Ask them to help you learn to forgive and forget.

3. Journal and pray about it.

4. Make a plan to grow in forgiveness and freedom.

5. Once you are free from the offense by learning to forgive, encourage others by sharing your story and teaching that forgiveness leads to freedom.

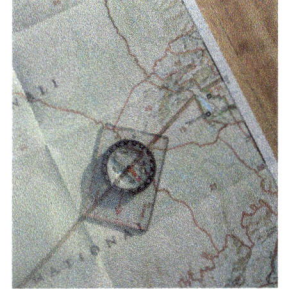

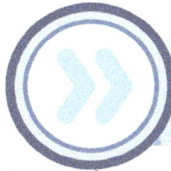

APPLICATION:

Learning to forgive is learning to let go of the hurt or offense forever. If you say you've forgiven someone and you are still holding a grudge, you are not forgiving them. First, write the name of the person who offended you, on a piece of paper (like an IOU). Then fold it up. Quietly say, "I choose to forgive (name the person and the offense). Finally, tear up the piece of paper and/or burn it, symbolizing that their debt, their IOU, is canceled forever.

Remind yourself that you've canceled their debt, and don't go digging in the trash and pick it up again. Move on with life and enjoy your freedom. Watch how the pain, shame, hurt and resentment go away as you truly forgive others in your heart.

Personal Follow-Up Activities and Ideas:

- Spend some time journaling
- Write your own poem or story
- Take a hike and think on it
- Share your thoughts with others
- Write a song.

- Create a drama, illustration or game
- Make your own video
- Start a positive group or club
- Create a related art project
- Or do something inspired just by you!

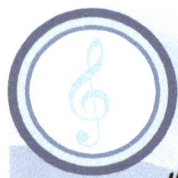

SONGS TO TAKE YOU HIGHER

"Rise Up Mighty Warrior" by Broken Walls

"I Forgive You" by Kellie Pickler

"Forgive Yourself" by Inna Modja

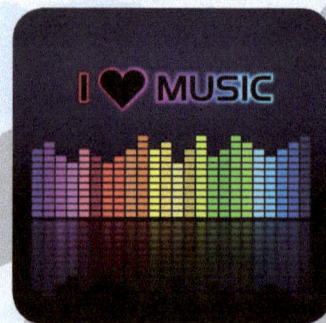

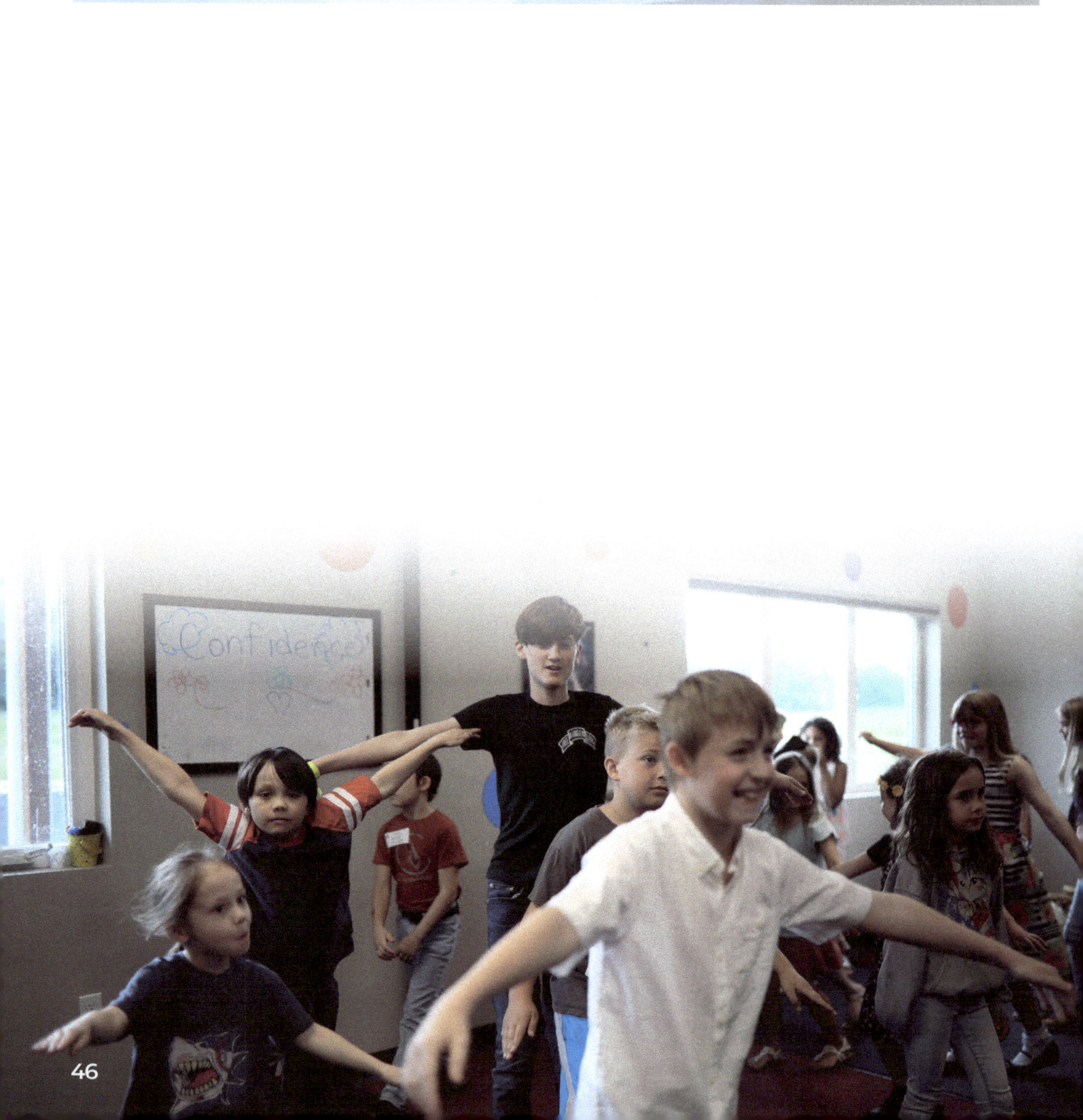

I ♥ MUSIC

RISE ABOVE IT!

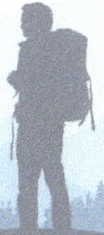

STRENGTH TO CLIMB

SUBJECT:
INNER STRENGTH/NOT GIVING UP

Written by Lyon Kopsak (Yuyanq' Ch'ex Team Member)

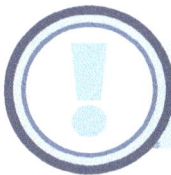

ATTENTION GETTERS

💬 QUOTES & THOUGHT SHOTS:

A. "It is not the critic who counts; not the man who points out how the strong man stumbles, or where the doer of deeds could have done them better. The credit belongs to the man who is actually in the arena, whose face is marred by dust and sweat and blood; who strives valiantly; who errs, who comes short again and again, because there is no effort without error and shortcoming; but who does actually strive to do the deeds; who knows great enthusiasms, the great devotions; who spends himself in a worthy cause; who at the best knows in the end the triumph of high achievement, and who at the worst, if he fails, at least fails while daring greatly, so that his place shall never be with those cold and timid souls who neither know victory nor defeat." ~ *Theodore Roosevelt*[1]

B. "Never let yourself get tired of doing good; in time it will pay off !" ~ *Amanda Pagaran*

C. "There is a secret to endure (and even be content) in any situation; you will discover it if you look." ~ *Amanda Pagaran*

D. "Some of the best lessons we ever learn we learn from our mistakes and failures. The error of the past is the wisdom and success of the future." ~ *Tyron Edwards*[2]

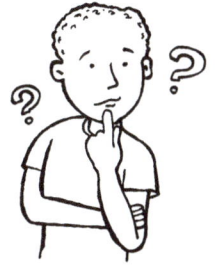

👁 VIDEO CLIP:

Kung Fu Panda | Today is a Gift[3] ▶ *https://youtu.be/BwqSraJpqfs*

🗣 DISCUSSION:

1. What did you learn from the *Kung Fu Panda* movie clip about perspective (or how to look at life)?

2. How does your perspective change what you choose to do?

3. Have you ever felt like you're not good enough?

4. Who helped Po (the panda) when he felt like a failure?

5. Who can you go to for help when you feel like you're not good enough or want to give up?

6. Why can spending energy regretting the past or worrying about the future hinder your progress?

7. What did the old wise one mean when he said, "Today is a gift; that is why it is called the Present"?

8. What else did you learn from this that might help you?

ACTIVITIES

GAME: Human Knot (Dr. Untangle)

Materials: *None*

Messy Rating: Low

Duration: *10 to 15 minutes*

Cost: *$0*

Have a group of 5 to 15 students stand very close together in a circle, except for one person who sits out for now. Have them reach into the center so all hands are jumbled and intertwined. Tell them to grab two other hands, one with each one of their own hands (but not a hand of the person next to them). Ensure that each person grabs two hands from two different people. Now they are a human knot. Without talking, and without letting go of any hands, they must use teamwork to untangle themselves into one large circle (Sometimes it's actually two or three circles).

As they progress, if they do not give up and let go of hands, you can make the task easier by increments. Below are some great ideas on how to, little by little, reward them for their persistence by making it a bit easier:

After a while...

1. Let the person who sat out, come over and use motions and pointing to "advise" them, but without talking.

2. Let the adviser speak.

3. Let everyone speak.

4. Let the group choose one set of hands that will be allowed to let go for a few seconds to be readjusted.

5. The teacher/leader can step in and help any way he/she sees fit.

After the activity, discuss results: What did they learn that will help them be better at it next time? How were they rewarded for not giving up? In what ways can it be similar to "not giving up" in real life? Note that even when it seems failure is inevitable, when people continue to press ahead, positive things can happen.

The Lesson: *Fail, learn, keep moving ahead.*

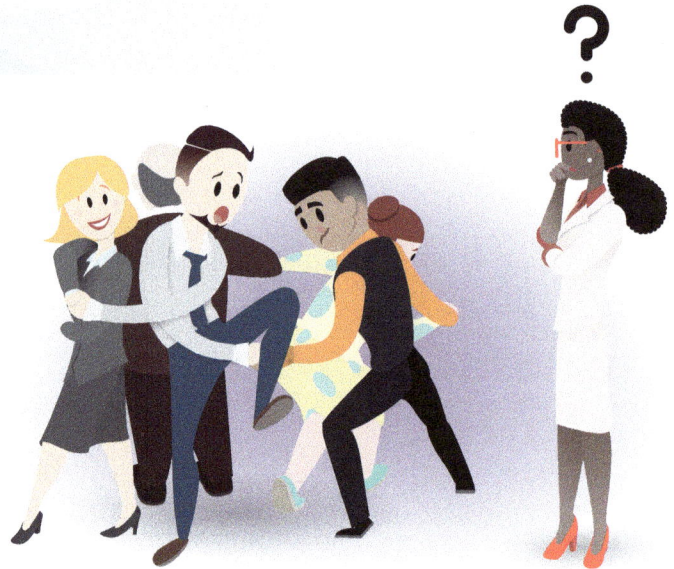

LESSON

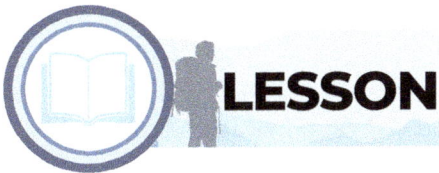

What Do Others Who Have Learned to Rise Above It Say?

LYON KOPSAK:

True inner strength is rising above. It can be rising above failure, disappointment, rejection, or any number of setbacks. Sometimes these setbacks are our fault, and sometimes they're not. Regardless, these moments can seem overwhelming.

All of us can look back at challenging moments in our lives—times when we've slipped and fallen—and remember how hard it was to get back up. If we've experienced this and moved past whatever it was that knocked us down, it means we're developing inner strength. Think of a time when you were at a low point in life but found the strength to continue.

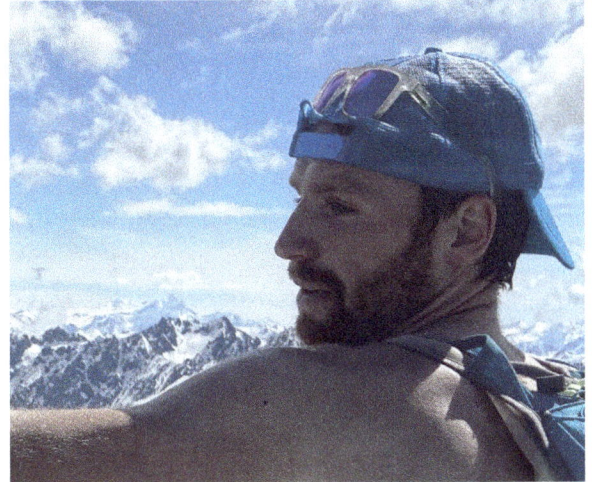

What if these seemingly overwhelming obstacles are opportunities? Opportunities to learn, to become stronger, to become more resilient. It's easy to feel down, hopeless, and uninspired after a setback, but really, these are crucial moments in our journey. Rising above obstacles defines who we are and makes us stronger.

It is essential to keep this perspective. Surround yourself with encouraging people in your life (parents, friends, teachers, coaches) who can inspire you and can reinforce this truth. Our lives have a purpose. Challenges in our lives have a purpose. Believing that everything can be done by ourselves and with our own strength leads to disappointment and discouragement. Always remember that failure is not final.

LYON'S PERSONAL EXPERIENCE:

I learned that failure and setbacks are important opportunities, and are just as important as success. Like many people, I tried at first to rely exclusively on my own strength. It only led to failure and disappointment. It is vital to have a positive response in these situations, and to reach out to others.

One example of this came during my senior year in high school. Life was going well and I felt like I could do anything. I had narrowed my college choices to three schools and was very confident that I would be accepted. It worked out that I received my acceptance notifications from the three schools all on the same day. All three schools turned me down. I felt like a complete failure. I was discouraged and embarrassed. I was supposed to be the guy who could do anything.

I did not feel like moving past this setback in my life. I had put all my hope into getting accepted into those schools. I was in desperate need of encouragement and support. I ended up turning to my family and friends. It wasn't fun, but because I had support from other people in my life, I was able to move past this obstacle. My family helped with the logistics of determining other feasible options for college. My friends helped by reminding me of all the things I had to be thankful for. It didn't take me long to regain perspective, get accepted into a different school, and continue my journey.

Looking back on what at the time felt like failure, I wouldn't change anything. I ended up in a school that shaped who I am today. Not only did I graduate, but I was also able to compete as an athlete during my time there. This would have been unlikely had I gotten into those other schools. When one door closed in my life, two more opened, and they were great doors.

Remember, our lives have a purpose. Setbacks and failure have a purpose. Surround yourself with trusted people who can reinforce a positive perspective. When you get knocked down, get back up.

HEROES WHO LEARNED TO BE RESILIENT

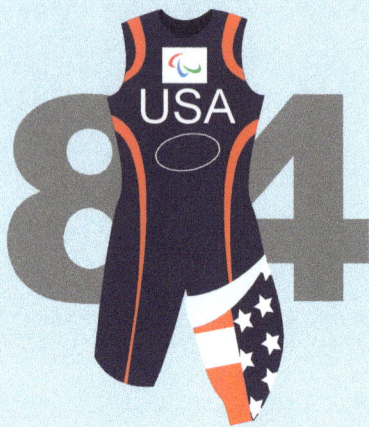

Melissa Stockwell is a wife, mom, Purple Heart recipient, and Paralympic athlete. Melissa lost one of her legs while serving in the military; she was 24 at the time. Four years later she was competing in the 2008 Paralympic games, and in 2016, she won a bronze medal.[4] Melissa experienced a significant setback and her journey has been full of challenges. She attributes her ability to move forward to people who have helped and encouraged her, as well as her choice to focus on the present. Learn more by reading her book *The Power of Choice: My Journey from Wounded Warrior to World Champion* or visiting her website:

🌐 *https://melissastockwell.com*

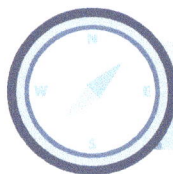

GPS: *WHAT PATH OR TRAIL DO I TAKE*

When you experience adversity, setbacks and challenges:

1. Share your experience with your mom, dad, a grandparent, or trusted elder.
2. Share your experience with your school counselor, teacher, pastor, priest, coach, or friend.
3. Remember past times when you've endured and overcome.
4. Remember that your life and these experiences have a purpose.
5. Make a plan, learn from your situation, and never give up hope.
6. Once you have risen above, learn to encourage others by sharing your story

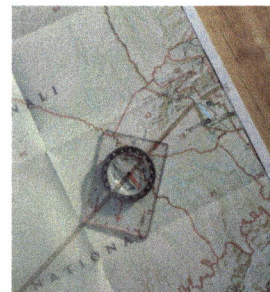

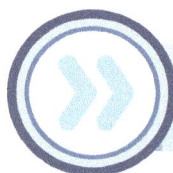

APPLICATION

PERSONAL FOLLOW-UP ACTIVITY IDEAS:

1. Discuss with a friend a time when you endured, stayed strong, tried again, or didn't give up and it paid off .
2. Journal about your thoughts about inner strength. What does it really mean?

3. Write a poem or song about having the strength to climb. Consider sharing it with someone who needs encouragement.

4. Take a hike and think about inner strength. Make some good goals and advance decisions concerning any future challenges that may arise.

5. Create a skit or drama that has a theme that teaches one of these lessons you've learned.

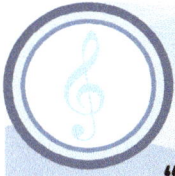

SONGS TO TAKE YOU HIGHER

"One Day" by Matisyahu

"I Can See Clearly Now" by Johnny Nash

"The Climb" by Miley Cyrus

"Brave" by Sara Bareilles

"You Make Me Brave" by Amanda Cook

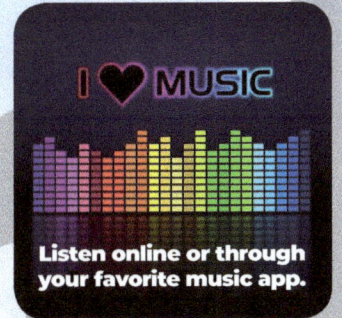

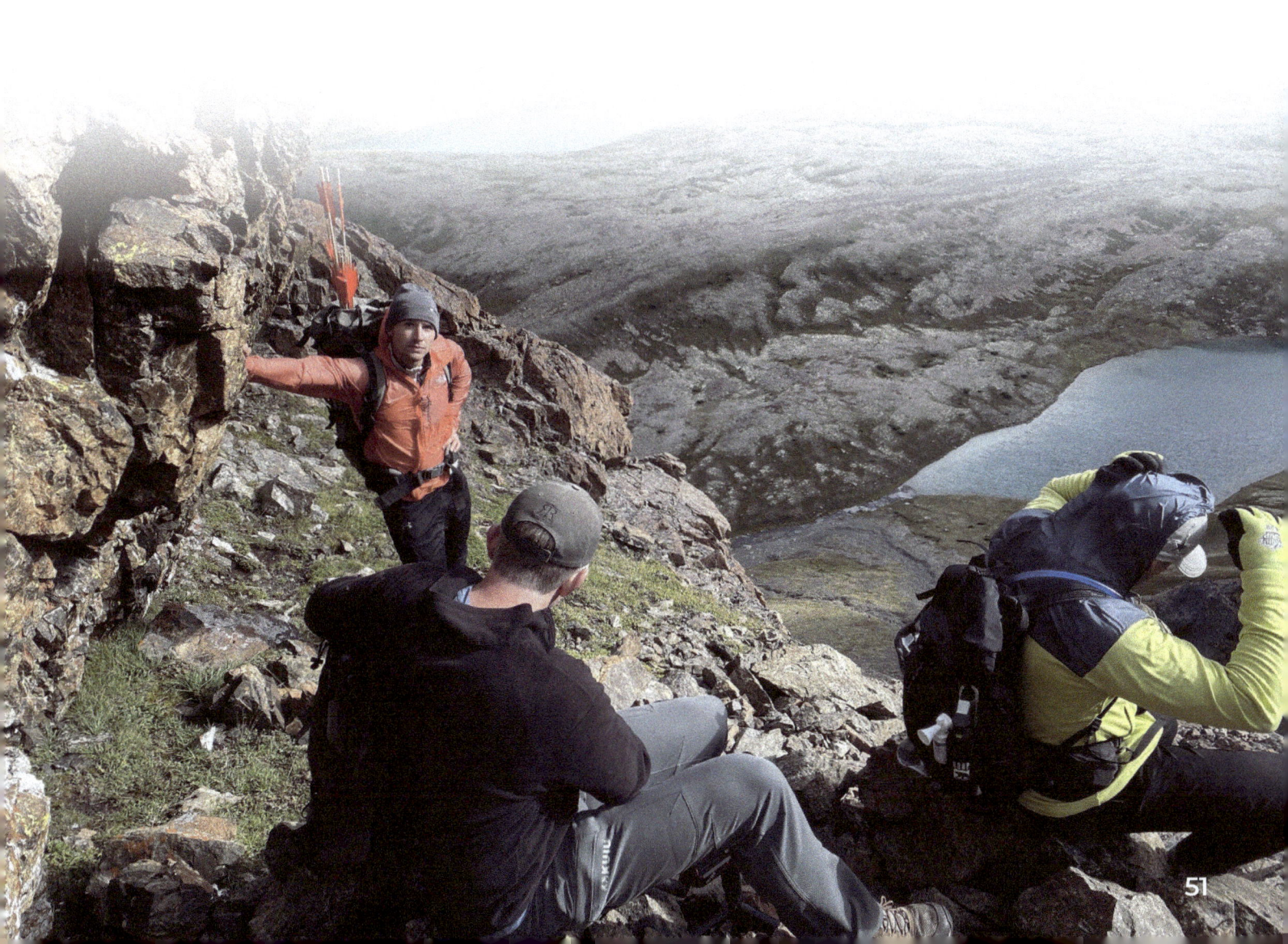

I ♥ MUSIC

Listen online or through your favorite music app.

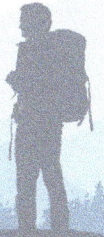

ASK FOR HELP
SUBJECT:
OVERCOMING DEPRESSION

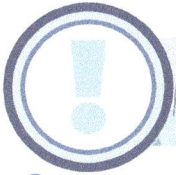

ATTENTION GETTERS

💬 QUOTES & THOUGHT SHOTS:

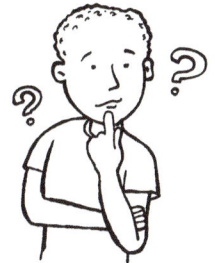

A. Don't continue to walk in darkness, turn on the light and watch the darkness run." ~ *Bill Pagaran*

B. "Depression is like a blanket of sadness and hopelessness that weighs us down and blinds us to our future. Ask for help removing it." ~ *Bill Pagaran*

C. "You were never meant to carry your burdens alone. People will always need people, and that's the way it should be." ~ *Amanda Pagaran*

D. "It makes others happy when they help you, so don't steal their blessing." ~ *Amanda Pagaran*

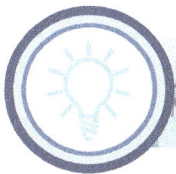

DEFINITION/INSIGHT:

FIVE REASONS WE SHOULD ASK FOR HELP

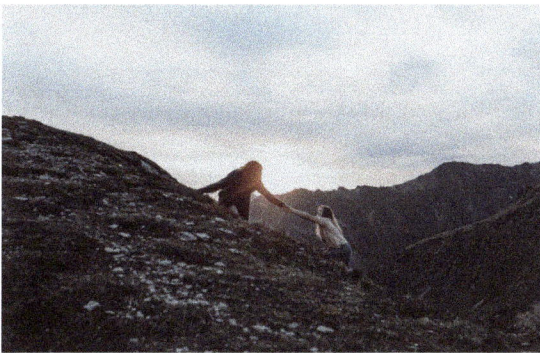

1. It connects you with others.
2. It builds courage to deal with rejection (builds resilience).
3. It increases your productivity.
4. It helps develop a mature mindset.
5. It makes you happy.

Think about the last time you asked for help. Did you feel thankful? Of course. And with research showing that people who [are thankful] are prone to experience more happiness and less anxiety, asking others for help, by extension, lets you achieve all these benefits.[1]

For a detailed version of the Five Reasons We Should Ask for Help More Often *by Jessica Gonzalez visit:*

🌐 *https://thriveglobal.com/stories/five-reasons-why-you-should-ask-for-help-more-often*

BLANKET GAME:

This activity is for teaching the importance of asking for help, but it is good if the leader lets the students problem-solve and figure that out on their own. During the second scenario, a few hints or some coaching may be necessary if the person under the blanket doesn't figure out to ask the other students for help.

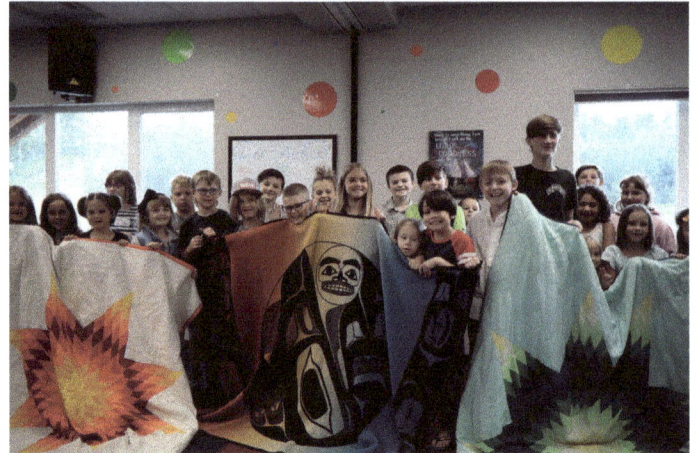

DIRECTIONS

Throw one or more oversized blankets over a volunteer who is seated cross-legged in the middle of the floor. (Make sure they won't be too hot, and that they'll be able to get enough air). Then quietly, without them knowing, place 4 to 8 chairs on top of the edges of the blanket(s). Have students sit in the chairs. Make sure that some of the chairs face in and some face out. (Secretly let those who are facing outward know that they should try to ignore what's going on in the circle until they have been asked three times to help or to co-operate by another chair-sitter. Those who face outward are not to respond directly to the person who is under the blanket.)

Try this activity with three scenarios.

SCENARIO #1:

The person under the blanket(s) tries to get out. They cannot use their hands *No one can talk.* (This usually fails, and after 5 to 10 minutes the leader can move on to Scenario #2.)

SCENARIO #2:

Reset the blanket(s), chairs, and positions of the players. (The leader may want to give a different volunteer the opportunity to be the one under the blanket this time.)

As before, the person under the blanket(s) tries to get out. They cannot use their hands, *but this time, everyone can talk.* As the person under the blanket realizes that they can ask for help from the other players, communication begins, and they can start to work as a team to solve the problem. (The leader can hint or coach them as needed if time passes and they are not realizing this.) Hopefully, the team will also realize that those with their backs to the center need special repeated prompting by the other chair-sitters in order to enlist their help, since the backwards-sitters are ignoring or unaware of the needs of the one under the blanket.

DISCUSSION

Before you reset the blanket(s), chairs and players for Scenario #3, discuss with the group the parallels between the activity and real-life situations in which they may need to ask for help, or in which they may need to help someone else.

1. Have you ever felt trapped in a bad situation, and maybe felt a little like the person under the blanket? Tell us about it? What was it like being trapped under a blanket?

2. Looking back at a time when you needed help, how were you "in the dark" about how to solve your problem?

3. How were you also in the dark or unaware of people around you who would want to help if you asked them, and could help you?

4. During that time in your life, or other tough times, how were your "hands tied" from being able to help yourself, and why did you feel you couldn't tell others about it or ask for help (like in the first scenario when the one under the blanket couldn't use hands or talk)?

5. Did you feel like some of those people around you were actually part of the problem (just like they were in the scenario, because they were sitting on the blanket that trapped you)? What could be done about those types of people?

6. Why do you think some people in the scenario were placed facing outward; and why do you think they had been instructed to ignore, or be unaware of, the person trapped underneath the blanket? *If they don't figure it out on their own, it is important that the leader helps them understand that not everyone in their lives will notice they need help, and there may even be some who don't care or are a detriment. However, if the student will keep asking for help, then others who do care and who do notice can all join together with you to enlist the help of experts or others who were unaware at first. The team can also work to get those who were in the way to cooperate better or to get out of the way.*

7. Why is it important to keep asking for help?

8. Next time you are feeling helpless, hopeless or in a bad situation, what can you do?

9. If you notice someone else who is in need of help, what are some things you can do? *The leader should encourage them to work with the person in need, to ask the right people for help, and to even form a team to problem-solve and work together the next time they know someone in need.*

SCENARIO #3: _____

Reset the blanket(s), chairs and players as in the first two scenarios. This third scenario is optional, but it can be an awesome concluding role play. This time, the leader can freely coach everyone in the scenario to communicate in positive, encouraging ways to cooperate and free the person from under the blanket(s). However, the leader should step back and be quiet if the students learned well from the discussion and are eagerly communicating in positive ways without prompting; in this way they'll gain confidence in their new skills and will experience the power they have to help others.

Afterward, let them reflect aloud about how it went this time compared to the first two times. Let them discuss what they learned. Note how much quicker, smoother, kinder, and even warmer it was this time through. Students are likely to end this activity feeling more relaxed and even joyful as they appreciate the interactions and relationships with one another that resulted from working effectively together to help someone.

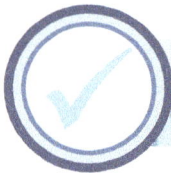

✓ JUST THE FACTS: *STATISTICS*

- Depression is the leading cause of disability in the United States among people ages 15 through 44.

- 80 percent of those treated for depression show signs of improvement within four to six weeks of starting treatment.

- Depression is treatable, and suicide is the most preventable type of death. Learning how to ask someone if they need help can save a life.

- According to the QPR Institute, "If people in a crisis get the help they need, they will probably never be suicidal again"[2]

HEROES WHO LEARNED TO BE RESILIENT

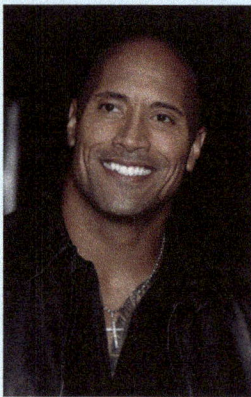

Dwayne "The Rock" Johnson, Katy Perry, Lady Gaga, Michael Phelps and many other celebrities struggled with severe depression and learned to overcome it and become successful in life. These celebrities learned to open up and talk about their hurt, pain and struggles. They also learned that they are not alone in their feelings. This led them to receive help and get back on track to pursue and achieve their dreams in life.

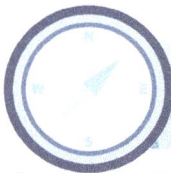

GPS: *WHAT DIRECTION DO I TAKE*

If you are feeling down, depressed or you need some help:

1. Talk to your mom, dad, grand-parent or trusted elder

2. Talk to a school counselor, teacher, pastor, priest or youth worker.

3. Take the Carry the Cure's Committed to Life Vow[3] (Promise to Live):
   🌐 *https://youtu.be/x-S_bS7FZcA*

4. Call one of these numbers:
   a. Alaska Care line: 1-877-266-4357
   b. Alaska 211
   c. AK State line (based out of Fairbanks, 24/7): 877-266-4951
   d. National Suicide Prevention Hotline (24/7): 1-800-273-8255
   e. Textline: Text "help" to 741741

5. Visit the Carry the Cure resource page: 🌐 *http://www.carrythecure.org/resource.html*

6. Journal and pray about it.

7. Make a plan to grow in forgiveness and freedom (see Rise Above It lesson, *Freedom in Forgiveness*).

8. Once you are free from the offense, learn to encourage others by sharing your story.

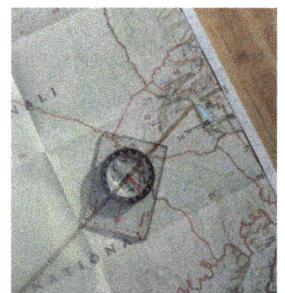

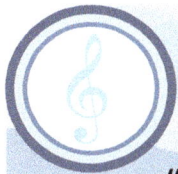 # APPLICATION

Talk to your parents, grandparents, trustworthy family members or friends about your dreams, struggles and challenges in life. Make it a regular event. I have a weekly group meeting and several weekly hikes that I go on with friends. During these meetings, I am able to share my fears, struggles, and dreams with people I trust. If darkness is beginning to weigh me down, these men and women are there to help remove that burden. They encourage me. They pray for me. They let me know they are there when I need them. Because of their faithful friendship and kindness, I'm comfortable in reaching out to them when I'm in need. Smile and show kindness to others who are going through tough times. Sometimes, the simple things like listening to others, showing kindness and a smile can make all the difference between life and death.

Personal Follow-Up Activity Ideas:

1. Spend time journaling about your thoughts.
2. Write a poem or story.
3. Take a hike and think about it.
4. Share your thoughts with others.
5. Write a song.
6. Create an illustration or game that has a theme of asking for help or intervention.
7. Make your own video.
8. Start a Positive Group or Club.
9. Create a related art project.
10. Create a skit or drama that has a theme that teaches one of these "lessons" you've learned.
11. Or do something inspired just by you!

SONGS TO TAKE YOU HIGHER

"Ride the Wind" by Broken Walls

"Fly" by Broken Walls

"Smile" by Uncle Kracker

"You Are Not Alone" by Meredith Andrews

"Alive" by P.O.D.

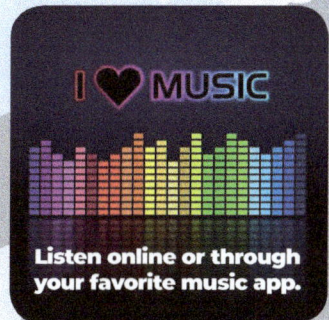

I ♥ MUSIC

Listen online or through your favorite music app.

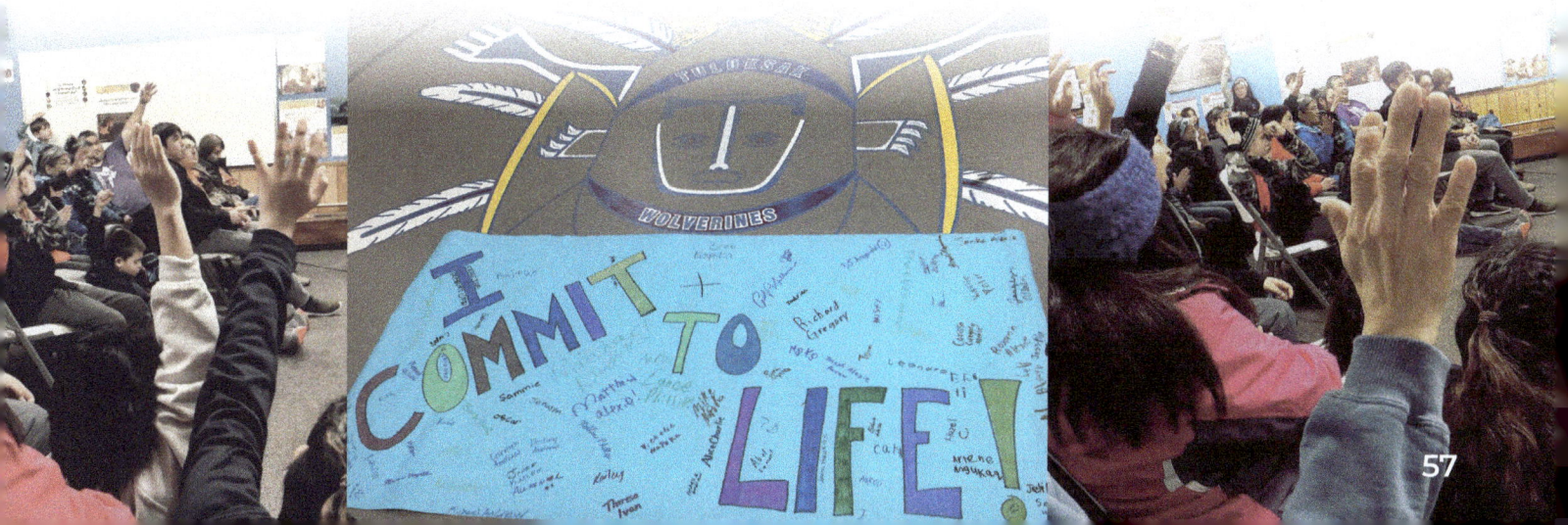

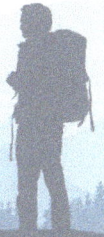

BOOMERANG

SUBJECT:
RESILIENCE/THE ABILITY TO BOUNCE BACK

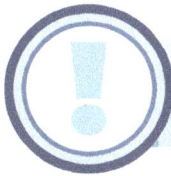 ## ATTENTION GETTERS

QUOTES & THOUGHT SHOTS:

A. Out of suffering have emerged the strongest souls; the most massive characters are seared with scars." ~ *Edwin H. Chapin*[1]

B. "Do not judge me by my success, judge me by how many times I fell down and got back up again." ~ *Nelson Mandela*[2]

C. "Those who can celebrate in the middle of a storm will often find they had reason to; and it sure makes the storm more fun." ~ *Amanda Pagaran*

D. "A rebound is underrated; it's usually in an upward direction, so look up!" ~ *Amanda Pagaran*

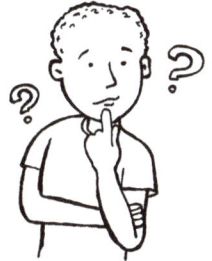

VIDEO CLIP:

JoJo Siwa - BOOMERANG (Official Video)[3] ▶ *https://youtu.be/ypPSrRYOAj4*

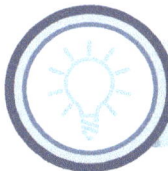 ## DEFINITION/INSIGHT

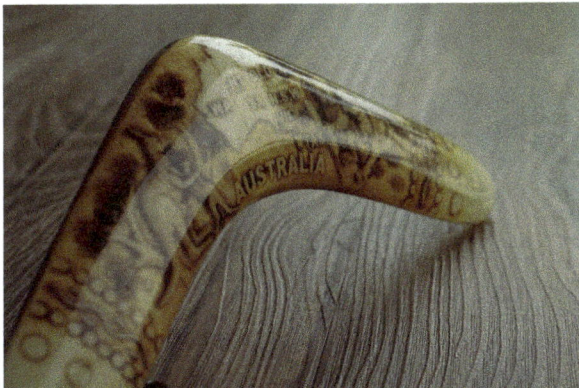

BOOMERANG:

A curved flat piece of wood that can be thrown so that it will return to the thrower, traditionally used by Australia's Aboriginal people as a hunting weapon.

Being resilient in life, can be compared to a boomerang.

RESILIENCE:

The capacity to recover quickly from difficulties; to bounce back.

Have students do a 5 to 6 minute free-write responding to the above quotes, video clip, and/or definition/insights. Have volunteers read some of their writings aloud. Follow with a class discussion reflecting on their related thoughts, reactions and ideas.

ACTIVITIES

GAME #1: Musical Chairs

Music: *Consider playing "Boomerang" by JoJo Siwa and other music with a positive message, for this game.*

This is an oldie, but a goodie, because one of the hardest lessons to learn when you're trying to build resiliency is that you don't always win—but that it's okay. Start the game by having the same number of chairs as players, so that everyone has a seat the first round. Then round by round, remove a chair each time so there will always be one child out (who finds no chair) when the music stops. Kids may experience emotions connected to becoming the odd one out and learn how to cope with those feelings.[4] Talk about it at the end of the game so students get a chance to express what they're experiencing, rather than just internalizing it.

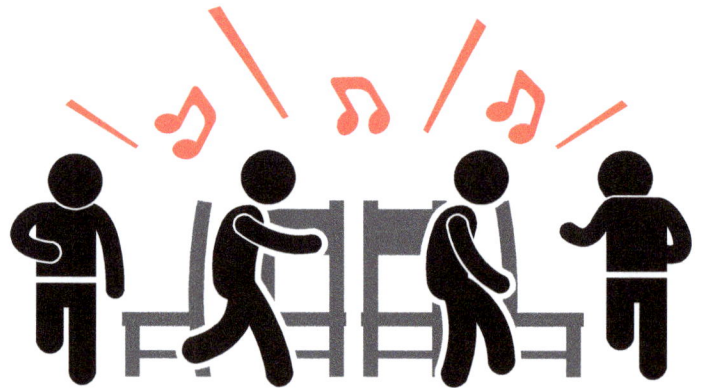

DISCUSSION: MUSICAL CHAIRS

1. How did you feel when the music stopped and there was no chair for you to sit in?
2. How did you feel when you had to watch others do what you once enjoyed?
3. Were there others still left in the game who you felt you could encourage and "cheer-on"?
4. How could you support others when they got left out?
5. Next time you play, can you think of strategies that might help you get farther?
6. Next time you play, can you think of ways to stay happy, positive, and help make the game fun for others?
7. How does this game relate to being resilient?

GAME #2: Hula-Hoop Challenge

Have the kids form a circle while holding hands, but before the last pair connect, place a hula-hoop over one arm. Without letting each other's hands go, the challenge is to get the hula-hoop to move around the circle. Students will have to work together to move the hoop and support each other so they don't fall over as they step through it.[4] After the game, follow-up with the following discussion.

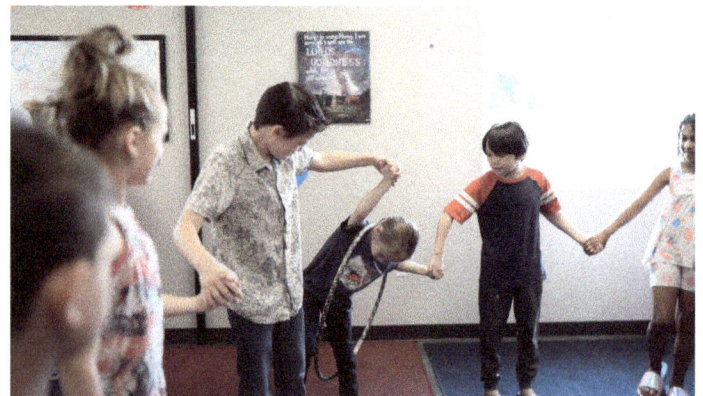

DISCUSSION: *HULA-HOOP GAME*

Another step towards building resiliency is learning to face conflict and develop problem-solving skills. Everything from picture puzzles to video games can teach problem solving and reasoning to students on their own, but it's also important to learn how to work with others to solve problems as a team. This game gives students a chance to work together, as a group, toward a common goal.

1. When the hula hoop came your way, how did you feel? Anxious or excited?
2. Did you welcome the challenge?
3. What made it difficult?
4. Did you listen to advice from other students about how to get through this challenge?
5. Did you ever feel stuck?
6. Did you fall or fail?
7. Did others make fun of you or help you? Did you help others?
8. What are some ideas you came up with to solve problems?
9. How can you relate this to going through personal challenges in life?
10. What kind of input would you value when in a tough situation in life?
11. How can you help others through their difficult times?

> For more games on building resilience see the following website:
> *https://www.tomsofmaine.com/good-matters/healthy-feeling/building-resilience-in-children-using-fun-games*

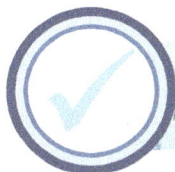

JUST THE FACTS: *STATISTICS*

According to Donald Meichenbaum, Ph.D, research indicates that half to two-thirds of children living in extreme circumstances (for example, homes where the caregivers struggle with addiction) grow up and overcome the odds and go on to achieve successful and well-adjusted lives.[5]

Also, according to the Mayo Health Clinic, resilience helps to protect from anxiety and depression.[6] Learn the benefits of resilience:

https://www.mayoclinic.org/tests-procedures/resilience-training/in-depth/resilience/art-20046311

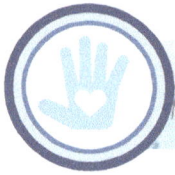

THOUGHTS FROM THE TEAM

Jonathan Maracle

Jonathan Maracle, the musician who wrote and performed the background song in the Rise Above It video *Ride the Wind* is a well-known Native American leader, songwriter, and the band leader of Broken Walls. He is half Mohawk and half Scottish. Growing up he was bullied by both Natives and non-Natives. He learned how to heal from all of the hurt and pain of his past, and even grow from it.

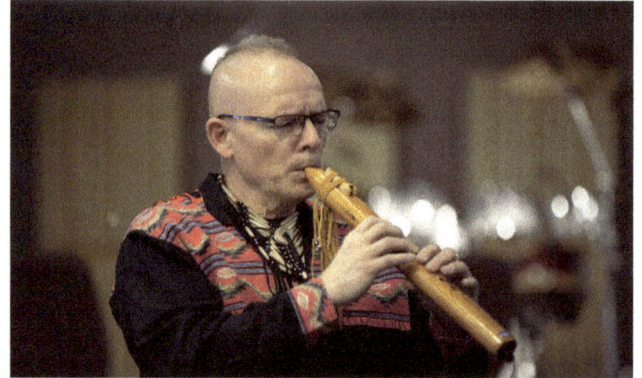

He learned how to love natives and non-natives. Now he leads one of the most effective organizations with the primary purpose of helping people reconcile their differences. He has helped thousands of people, both Native and non-Native, find peace with each other, and has given them tools to work together for healthier communities. He and his team have taught thousands of people how to break down the walls that separate them.

Most of the music of Broken Walls is focused on how to bring peace into difficult situations. Visit: ⊕ www.brokenwalls.com

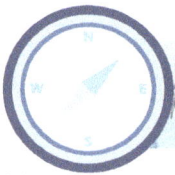

GPS: *WHAT DIRECTION DO I TAKE*

How can you build resilience in your life?

1. Get involved in group activities or clubs to learn how to work through challenges together.

2. Join a sport to learn the benefits of teamwork. Remember, there's no "I" in team.

3. Journal and pray about it.

4. When people put you down or tease you; learn how to reject hurtful comments and unhelpful opinions. Opinions are not fact. Learn how to rise above opinions and lies with truth.

5. Take it a step farther; if they put you down, learn how to speak life, encouragement and acceptance over them. It may not be instant, but watch how your attitude changes their heart and shapes their words from harmful to helpful. Also, note how you grow and mature as you learn how to encourage others.

6. Find a parent, family member, mentor, life coach, teacher, advisor, counselor, pastor, youth worker, or elder who can help build you up through life's challenges so you can learn how to bounce back to a healthy place in life whenever you have to face negative challenges.

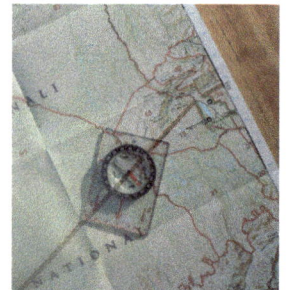

APPLICATION

You were born to come back, like a boomerang. You can be strong and resilient. You can learn from the toughest challenges in life. Whether hurtful words or a painful situation, there is always a way to heal, learn, grow stronger, and help others. That's one reason it is so important to find family and friends who will help you to learn how to bounce back.

Surround yourself with people who speak life. Find people who speak hope. Let those words of life and hope build up in your heart and fill you up. Don't make room in your heart and mind for things that will bring you down. Clothe yourself with armor in your heart and mind so that you do not accept the harmful things that others do or say. Model your life after others who don't repay evil with revenge; model your life after those who know the power of replacing evil with good. If people speak bad things over your life, say or do kind/positive things that replace the bad with good.

If you surround yourself with good role models, they can help you walk through those tough challenges in your life. Sometimes, you are given life lessons through constructive criticism. Those are words that are meant to correct us for good reasons. (Examples: Don't smoke, don't drink or use drugs, because they always lead to a path of destruction in life, or If you practice/rehearse more, your performance will improve.) Knowing how to apply them will help you grow as a healthy person. Learn the difference between mean words and constructive ones. Knowing the source can help you determine that.

Never give up, there's always hope! There are always others who have gone through whatever challenge you are facing, others who learned to thrive and not dive, and who eventually succeeded. They learned that the best things in life are worth fighting for. Your dreams, your goals and your future are worth it.

Personal Follow-Up Activities and Ideas:

- Spend some time journaling
- Write your own poem or story
- Take a hike and think on it
- Share your thoughts with others
- Write a song.

- Create a drama, illustration or game
- Make your own video
- Start a positive group or club
- Create a related art project
- Or do something inspired just by you!

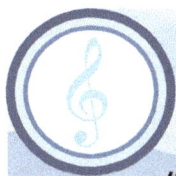

SONGS TO TAKE YOU HIGHER

"The Comeback" by Danny GoKey

"Boomerang" by JoJo Siwa

"Firework" by Katy Perry

"Headphones" by Britt Nicole

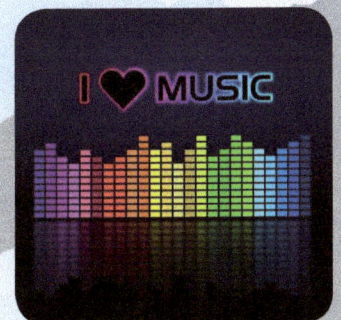

I ♥ MUSIC

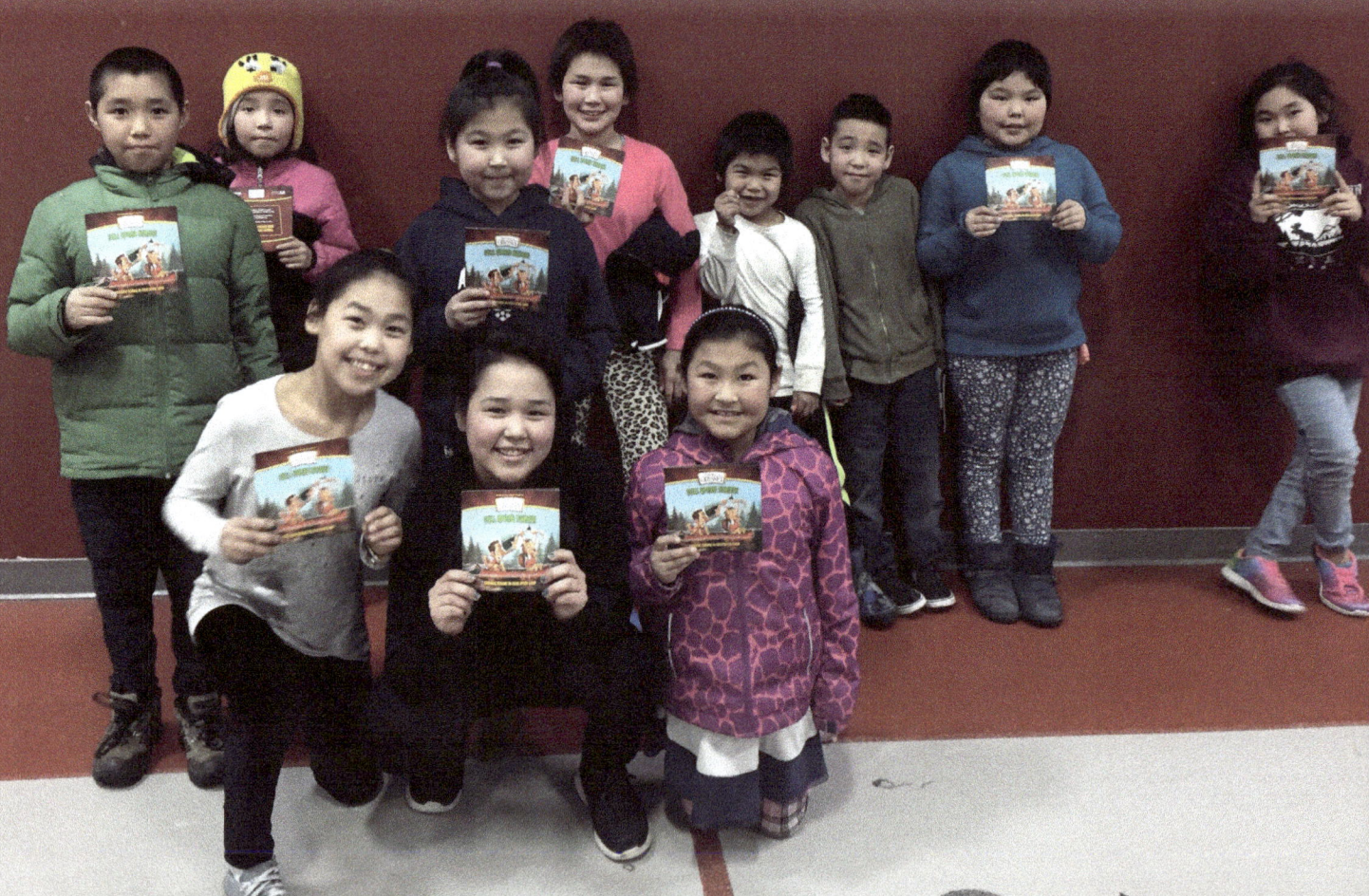

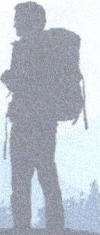

BETTER TOGETHER

SUBJECT:
UNITY

"Thoughts From the Team" and "Follow-Up" written by Jonathan Maracle

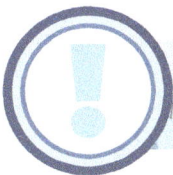

! ATTENTION GETTERS

💬 QUOTES & THOUGHT SHOTS:

A. "We must learn to live together as brothers, or perish together as fools."
   ~ *Martin Luther King*[1]

B. "We are better together." ~ *Anonymous*

C. "Even the weak become strong when they are united."
   ~ *Friedrich von Schiller*[2]

D. "For the strength of the Pack is the Wolf, and the strength of the Wolf is the Pack."
   ~ *Rudyard Kipling*[3]

E. "United we stand. Divided we fall." ~ *Patrick Henry*[4]

F. "We must, indeed, all hang together or, most assuredly, we shall all hang separately."
   ~ *Benjamin Franklin*[5]

G. "All for one and one for all!" ~ *Alexandre Dumas (The Three Musketeers)*[6]

H. "Treat others with love, because we all need others to lean on." ~ *Amanda Pagaran*

I. "Just like an apple on a tree, you cannot survive alone. The apple must be connected to the tree for survival, just as you must be 'connected' to survive. What do you call an independent apple? Either rotting or just plain eaten!" ~ *Amanda Pagaran*

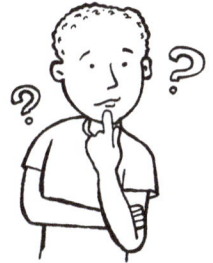

👁 VIDEO CLIP:

2011 LifeLight Festival: Broken Walls
▶ *https://youtu.be/pt-XpZlrTes*

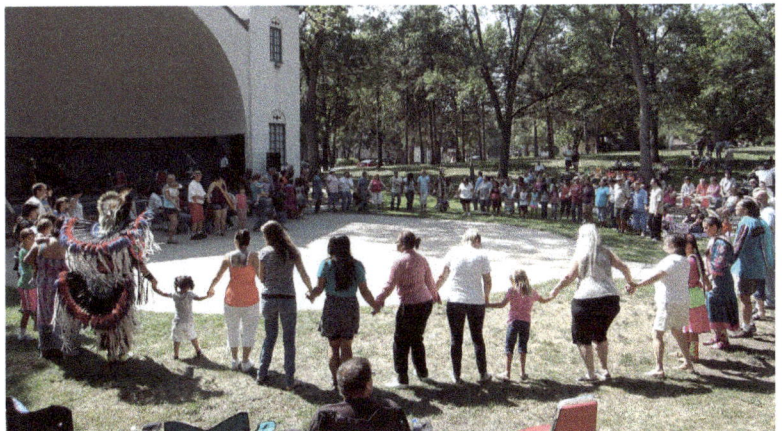

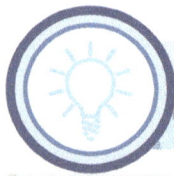

DEFINITION/INSIGHT

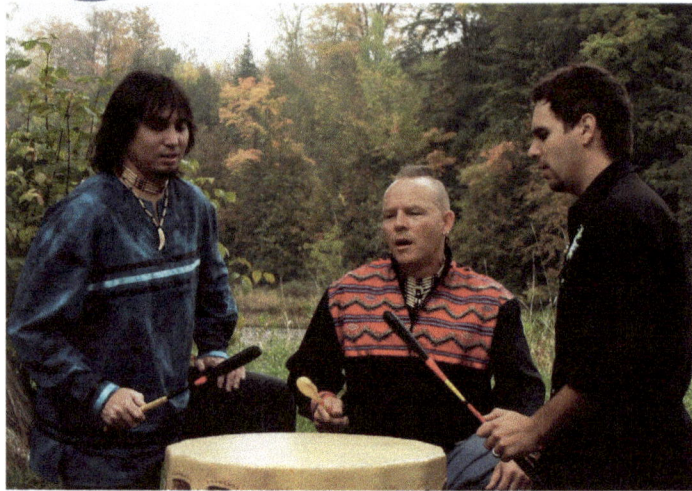

UNITY:

Unity is being together or being at one with someone or something. It's the opposite of being divided.

Unity is a word for togetherness or oneness. When a Native American drum group sits at the drum at a powwow, they play in unity. When the North won the Civil War, it assured the unity of the United States. Sports teams wear uniforms to show unity, and their fans wear team colors for the same reason. When a bunch of people act as one and are on the same page, they're displaying unity. When people are bickering and disorganized, there's no unity. In any group or cause, it takes work to find and maintain unity.

The Native American Round (Friendship) Dance gives the perfect visual of what unity looks like.

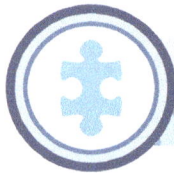

ACTIVITIES

GAME #1: Round Dance (Friendship Dance)

1. Explain why Native Americans do Round Dances: "As with many social dances, Round Dances foster pride and a sense of community amongst participants, renewing relationships with one another while celebrating First Peoples' identity." *~ Anna Hoefnagels (**Cree Round Dances**)*

   Examples of Alaska Native friendship dances include those done by the Yupik and Tlingit people. The Tlingit dances include a Call Out dance, in which they call each tribe out to dance (one at a time), in order to honor them. It culminates with everyone dancing to demonstrate unity.

2. Choose a song to play during your Round Dance.

   A. "Friendship Dance" by Broken Walls ⊕ *https://youtu.be/I4qbFSV_0_E*

   B. "Circle of the Creator" by Broken Walls ⊕ *https://youtu.be/ecXynVkWb4k*

   C. "Wave" by Broken Walls ⊕ *https://youtu.be/YTjTigRBwLl*

3. Have them do a round dance:

   A. Dancers join hands to form a large circle.

   B. Start the music.

   C. Everyone moves to their left , using a sideways shuffle-step on each beat, in-time with the long-short pattern of the drumbeats, and bending the knees slightly to bounce with each step. (The manner of the step, as well as the whole dance, can vary depending on the tribe. It's easiest to just have them copy the style used in the video clip you showed them.)

    D. Their grasped hands usually swing with each step. First forward, then back.

DISCUSSION:

One of the greatest leaders in our time, Loren Cunningham, says that there is beauty in diversity, because when we respect the people of the land, the different nations and cultures, then we honor Creator.

This inspires unity, which becomes a key to having a healed land and a healed people.

1. Recall a time in your past, (or if you can't think of one, maybe a scene from a show or movie) when failure or danger resulted because someone was alone. How might the story have ended differently if that person had been able and willing to unite with others?

2. Have you ever judged someone and later regretted it? Why?

3. In every Alaskan Native Traditional Values List, *respect* is one of the most important things. Why?

4. Do you have to like someone or agree with them to respect them?

5. Why does respect have to do with actions rather than feelings?

6. What does it look like to respect someone?

7. What are some ways that respecting others within a group, creates unity?

8. Why is unity a good thing?

9. How does a traditional Round Dance, or friendship dance, model unity with others?

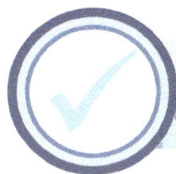

JUST THE FACTS (STATISTICS):

(Unity) Teamwork...

- Helps to reach a goal quicker
- Builds better friendships and better working relationships
- Helps us to better understand others
- Helps us get the job done right
- Promotes mutual respect and honor
- Motivates productivity in the workplace

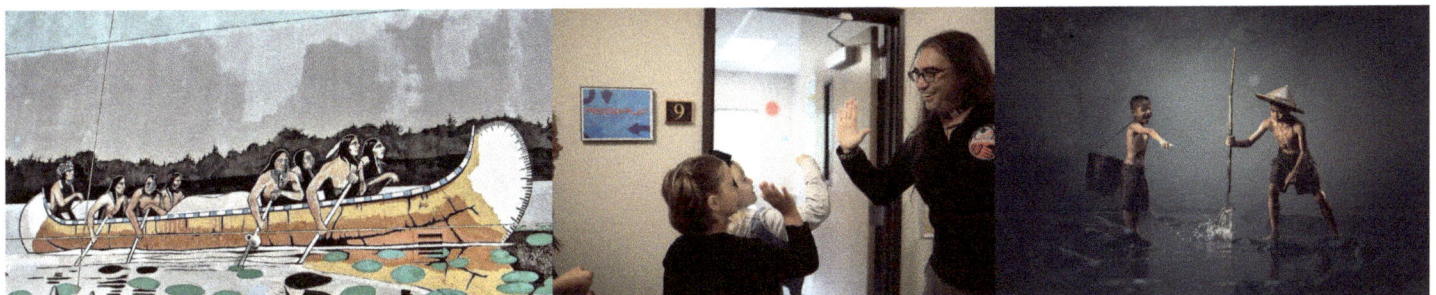

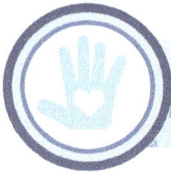

THOUGHTS FROM THE TEAM

Jonathan Maracle: *ON UNITY*

Seeking to bring unity is perhaps one of the most revealing aspects of who we are.

I have found that if I want to bring people together, I have to discover and embrace who I truly am. This reminds me of an old saying I heard years ago:

> ***"You must know who you are to know where you're going."***

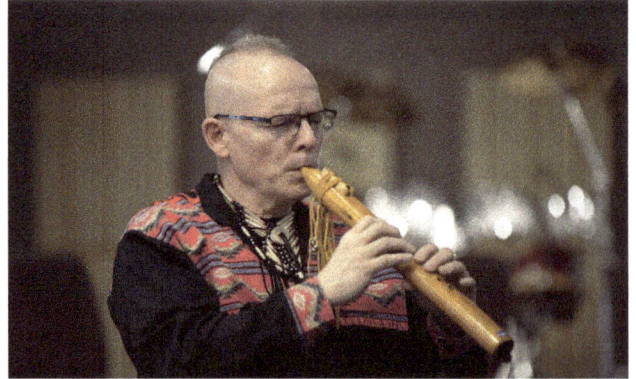

During my life, the people who have made the deepest impression on me are those who 1) **embrace who they are**, and 2) **realize their potential**. These two aspects of life are a good beginning and a foundation for success. I believe everyone was created with purpose, and when we seek, discover, and embrace this purpose it will ultimately lead us to bring unity and hope to those around us.

I found that to move forward exercising my gifts I had to look at the relationships I have had. Just like everyone else, I had to honestly decide which relationships I had handled well and which I had not. Then I had a choice: I had to decide how I was going to deal with past relationships as well as the new ones I would encounter.

These types of decisions are vital to the character-building one needs to bring unity. Decisions such as forgiving and being forgiven may sound simple, but when we decide to act on them, they reveal to us our personal inner battles that must be overcome to bring unity. Another example is pride. Be willing to recognize if pride is standing in the way of your success, and if so, then address it. Your choices are key.

> ***"You matter; the choices you make make a difference in the world around you."***

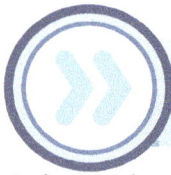

APPLICATION

Ask students what they have learned from the lesson today. How will it change any decisions they make in the future? How will it impact the way they treat others and interact with others? How will they demonstrate unity and show respect to those around them?

Personal Follow-Up Activities and Ideas: *FROM JONATHAN MARACLE*

Make your own personal list of things you do that are not productive in bringing unity. Recognize them when they are about to happen, make a commitment to yourself to stop doing them, and replace them with something that will bring unity.

Your list needs to start with changes you want to make in your personal life. Then expand it to all aspects of your life.

FIRST, CONSIDER: You, your personal thought life, and your actions

NEXT, CONSIDER: Your thought life and interactions within your family

FINALLY, CONSIDER: Your thought life and interactions with others outside your family

Then act!

Don't put off the things you know you need to do. So many people have great thoughts and ideas, but we must act to see progress. Be the catalyst for positive change. Put your good thoughts and words into action.

As a songwriter I have learned that I must act when the song inspiration is there. Sometimes I'm tired and I just don't feel like writing down the ideas, but when I act and embrace the moment, those embraced moments turn into songs. We can apply this principle to life, so embrace the moment and act, and become a powerful unifying source for everyone around you!

Always remember...

"Be yourself and change the world!"

Here are the lyrics to a song I have written; I hope it can be an encouragement to you.

I SEE BEAUTY
Written by Jonathan Maracle Socan, 1999

We all have a purpose, each one plays a part
The path that you walk on, let it be
Let it be the right one

I see beauty, when I see you
The gifts you share and the color of your skin
As we give of ourselves, we make life so much sweeter
And through honor a better place to live
Through honor a better place to live

We celebrate the fall of the wall
And the joy of coming together
We see the hope of how things could be
And the change when we're together
And the change when we're together

Respond with your gift, as a matter of your heart
One step at a time, is a good place to start

I see beauty, the difference between us
The gifts you share and the color of your skin
As we give of ourselves, we make life so much sweeter.
And the world a better place to live.
Through honor a better place to live.

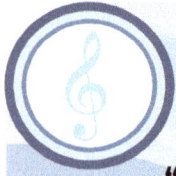

SONGS TO TAKE YOU HIGHER

"We're All In This Together" from High School Musical

"One Blood" by Jonathan Maracle

"We Are One" by Broken Walls

"Keep Changing the World" by Mikeschair

"With My Own Two Hands" by Ben Harper *(or Jack Johnson version)*

"Do Something" by Matthew West

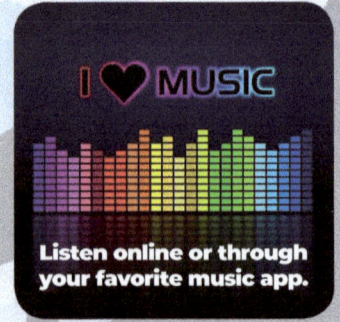

I ♥ MUSIC

Listen online or through your favorite music app.

RISE ABOVE IT!

CARRY THE CURE'S
COMMITTED TO LIFE VOW

I vow to commit to life and pursue my purpose.

Whether times are good or bad,

whether I have money or not;

even if I'm sick;

when I'm alone or lonely,

I CHOOSE LIFE!

When there's too much pressure;

or, when I've lost hope;

I'll ask for help.

I am valuable.

I am loved.

There's a good plan for my life.

I have a purpose.

I COMMIT TO LIFE!

Here's a YouTube video link to Carry the Cure's Committed to Life Vow. Use this when you want your group, class or people at your event to make this declaration of life.

https://youtu.be/x-S_bS7FZcA

RESOURCES

SUICIDE PREVENTION IS EVERYBODY'S BUSINESS.
YOU CAN HELP SAVE LIVES!

NEED HELP?

- Talk to a family member, friend, health care provider, teacher, elder, faith leader or counselor.

- Call your local mental health agency or crisis team.

- Text *CONNECT* to 741741.

- Call the *National Suicide Prevention Lifeline:* 1- 800-273-TALK (8255).

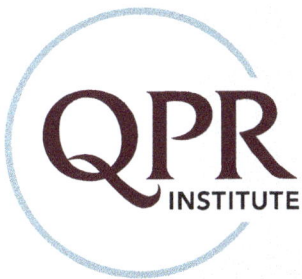

QPR INSTITUTE

LEARN HOW TO "ASK A QUESTION AND SAVE A LIFE."

QPR = **Q**uestion. **P**ersuade. **R**efer.
Three steps everyone can learn to save a life.

🌐 www.qprinstitute.com

CARELINE 1-877-266-4357

ALASKA'S SUICIDE PREVENTION AND SOMEONE TO TALK TO LINE

Feeling down or thinking of suicide?
Please know that you can feel better about yourself and your life.

For free, confidential help 24/7, call the Alaska Careline (1-877-266-4357) or text **4help** to 839863, from 3-11pm Tuesday-Saturday

Get the Careline App or visit their website: **https://carelinealaska.com**

NATIONAL

SUICIDE

PREVENTION

LIFELINE™

1-800-273-TALK (8255)

suicidepreventionlifeline.org

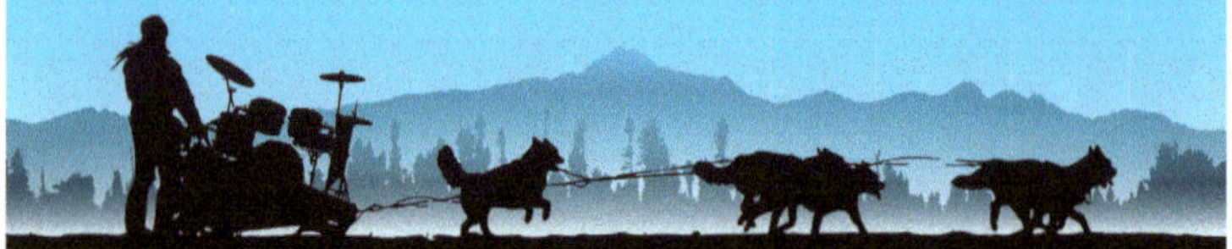

CARRY THE CURE

For more resources
visit Carry the Cure's website

https://carrythecure.org/resource.html

END NOTES
REFERENCES/SOURCES BY CHAPTER

How to Use This Book

1.   John 8:32

Chapter 1 - Light Up the World

1.   Pagaran, William. "Hope To Rise Above It!" YouTube - Hope To Rise Above. YouTube. Accessed October 23, 2021. https://www.youtube.com/watch?v=cn7JxtCIQzs.

2.   Carry The Cure, Inc. "Carry The Cure: Resources." Carry the Cure, Inc. - Resource. Accessed October 23, 2021. http://www.carrythecure.org/resource.html.

3.   The Human Flourishing Program. Accessed October 23, 2021. https://hfh.fas.harvard.edu/.

4.   Enayati, Amanda. "How Hope Can Help You Heal | CNN." How hope can help you heal. CNN, April 11, 2013. https://www.cnn.com/2013/04/11/health/hope-healing-enayati/index.html.

5.   Temple, Mitch. "Restore Hope for Your Marriage." Focus on the Family, September 30, 2021. https://www.focusonthefamily.com/marriage/restore-hope-for-your-marriage/.

6.   "QPR Institute: Practical and Proven Suicide Prevention Training." QPR Institute | Practical and Proven Suicide Prevention Training QPR Institute (en-US). Accessed October 23, 2021. http://www.qprinstitute.com/.

7.   Davis, Paula. "5 Ways Hope Impacts Health & Happiness." Psychology Today. Sussex Publishers, March 3, 2013. https://www.psychologytoday.com/us/blog/pressureproof/201303/5-ways-hope-impacts-health-happiness.

8.   Acharya, Tanvia, and Mark Agius. "The Importance of Hope against Other Factors in the Recovery of Mental Illness." Psychiatria Danubina. U.S. National Library of Medicine, September 29, 2017. https://pubmed.ncbi.nlm.nih.gov/28953841.

9.   Yotsidi, V., A. Pagoulatou, T. Kyriazos, and A. Stalikas. "Open Journal of Social Sciences." The Role of Hope in Academic and Work Environments: An Integrative Literature Review, June 22, 2021. https://www.scirp.org/(S(i43dyn45teexjx455qlt3d2q))/reference/referencespapers.aspx?referenceid=3012672 .

10. Akita, Lailah Gifty. Think Great, Be Great! Seattle, WA: CreateSpace, 2015.

11. Christopher Reeve: Hope In Motion. USA: Virgil Films, 2007.

12. Meyer, Joyce. *Get Your Hopes Up!: Expect Something Good to Happen to You Every Day.* New York: Faith Words, 2016.

13. Amy. "57 Ways to Spread Kindness and Brighten a Day." Charity Ideas, October 26, 2011. https://charityideasblog.com/2011/10/26/57-ways-to-spread-kindness/ .

Chapter 2 - Check Your Tires & Keep Your Seatbelt On

·   Oliver Goldsmith - 1774 - Public Domain

1.   Farrell, Don. Essay. In The Good Book of Business: The Most Redeeming Book of Answers to Questions About Small Business Problems & Challenges, 1559. Minneapolis, MN: Publish Green, 2012.

2.   Issacson, Walter. Essay. In Einstein: His Life and Universe, 367. New York, NY: Simon & Schuster, 2007.

3.   Swanson, Jan, and Alan Cooper. A Physician's Guide to Coping with Death and Dying. Montreal, Ontario: McGill-Queen's University Press, 2005.

4.   "Rascal Flatts - Life Is a Highway." Accessed October 23, 2021. https://www.youtube.com/watch?v=5tXh_MfrMe0.

5.   Demientieff, Adam. "Four Man Carry WEIO 2012." Accessed October 23, 2021. https://www.youtube.com/watch?v=A7sJnuACWi4.

6.   Assess Your Health. Accessed October 23, 2021. https://www.drwalt.com/PDF/Assessyourhealth.pdf.

Chapter 3 - The Name Game

1.   Brown, Brené. The Gifts of Imperfection. Cheongha/ Tsai Fong Books. 2011.

2.   Brown, Brené. My Story Matters Because I Matter I Am Absolutely Enough. Empowered Publishers. 2019.

3.   Kennedy, Lou. Business Etiquette for the Nineties: Your Ticket to Career Success, 8. Palmetto Publishers. 1992.

4.   Rocky Balboa IV. DVD. USA: Metro-Goldwyn-Mayer, 1985.

5.   "Baby Names." SheKnows, August 13, 2020. https://www.sheknows.com/baby-names/.

6.   Russell, Joyce E.A. "Career Coach: The Power of Using a Name." The Washington Post, January 12, 2014. https://www.washingtonpost.com/business/capitalbusiness/career-coach-the-power-of-using-a-name/2014/01/10/8ca03da0-787e-11e3-8963-b4b654bcc9b2_story.html.

7.   "Lauren Daigle - You Say (Official Music Video) - Youtube." You Say. Accessed October 23, 2021. https://www.youtube.com/watch?v=slaT8Jl2zpl.

8.   "Katy Perry - Roar (Official) - Youtube." Accessed October 23, 2021. https://www.youtube.com/watch?v=CevxZvSJLk8.

Chapter 4 - Reach For The Heavens

1.   Center of the Storm. DVD. USA: Thirteen/WNET, 2002.

2. "There Are Some People Who Live in a Dream World, and There Are Some Who Face Reality and Then There Are Those Who Turn One into the Other." Douglas H. Everett: There are some people who live in a dream world, and there are some who face reality and then there are those who turn one into the other. Accessed October 23, 2021. https://www.quotes.net/quote/12897.

3. Marajulienne. "Prince's Speech - Compressed.mp." YouTube, March 31, 2012. https://bit.ly/3nQCPrq.

4. "Martin Luther King Jr's 'I Have a Dream' Speech." YouTube. MixedNationEnt, June 23, 2011. https://bit.ly/3q7vsxD.

5. https://www.mindwise.org/blog/community/the-power-and-science-of-hope/

6. "Harriet Tubman." Biography.com, A&E Networks Television, 11 Aug. 2021, https://www.biography.com/activist/harriet-tubman.

Chapter 5 - The Strength of a Good Friend

1. Carnegie, Dale. How to Win Friends & Influence People. Gallery Books, 2013.

2. Ziglar, Zig. Great Quotes from Zig Ziglar. Career Press, 1997.

3. "Ed Cunningham Quotes." Quotes.net. STANDS4 LLC, 2021. Web. 27 Dec. 2021. https://www.quotes.net/quote/12258.

4. Brisbaine, Authur. The Book of Today. International Magazine Company, 1923.

5. Maltz, Maxwell. Psycho-Cybernetics: Updated and Expanded. Perigee, an Imprint of Penguin Random House LLC, 2015.

6. Smith, Will. "Will Smith - Friend like Me (from Aladdin... - Youtube." Will Smith - Friend Like Me (from Aladdin) (Official Video), August 5, 2019. https://www.youtube.com/watch?v=1at7kKzBYxI.

7. "Caminandes3:Llamigos,"January29,2016.https://www.youtube.com/watch?v=SkVqJ1SGeL0.

8. Weng, Modern, and Meredith Bland. "Friendship Activities: 10 Top Games for Kids." Healthline, Healthline Media, 3 Nov. 2015, https://www.healthline.com/health/parenting/friendship-activities#Middle-School-Friendship-Activities.

9. Ditch The Label. "21 Facts about Bullying That You Probably Never Knew." Ditch the Label, 30 June 2021, https://www.ditchthelabel.org/21-facts-about-bullying/.

Chapter 6 - Freedom in Forgiveness

1. Smedes, Lewis B. Forgive and Forget: Healing the Hurts We Don't Deserve. New York, NYz: HarperOne, 2007.

2. Williamson, Marianne. "Marianne Williamson Quotes." BrainyQuote. Xplore. Accessed September 6, 2021. https://www.brainyquote.com/quotes/marianne_williamson_635346.

3. Batterson, Mark. "3 Questions: Mark Batterson." Guideposts, July 29, 2021. https://www.guideposts.org/inspiration/inspiring-stories/stories-of-faith/3-questions-mark-batterson.

4. "The Princess Bride (5/12) Movie Clip - Youtube," February 11, 2015. https://www.youtube.com/watch?v=rMz7JBRbmNo.

5. "Forgiveness: Your Health Depends on It." Johns Hopkins Medicine. Accessed September 1, 2021. https://www.hopkinsmedicine.org/health/wellness-and-prevention/forgiveness-your-health-depends-on-it.

Chapter 7 - Strength to Climb

1. 1. Roosevelt, Theodore. "The Man in the Arena." TR Center - The Man in the Arena, April 11, 2011. https://www.theodorerooseveltcenter.org/Blog/Item/The%20Man%20in%20the%20Arena.

2. EDWARDS, TRYON. New Dictionary of Thoughts - A Cyclopedia of Quotations from the Best Authors of the World, ... Both Ancient and Modern, Alphabetically Arranged B. Redditch, Worcestershire, UK: Read Books Ltd, 2011.

3. "Kung Fu Panda | Today Is a Gift - Youtube." Kung Fu Panda - Today Is A Gift. Best Movie Vines, August 17, 2017. https://www.youtube.com/watch?v=BwqSraJpqfs.

4. Stockwell, Melissa. "Melissa Stockwell." Melissa Stockwell | Home, December 11, 2018. https://melissastockwell.com/.

Chapter 8 - Ask For Help

1. Gonzalez, Jessica. "Five Reasons Why You Should Ask for Help More Often." Thrive Global, February 26, 2020. https://thriveglobal.com/stories/five-reasons-why-you-should-ask-for-helpmore-often/.

2. Paul Quinnett, Ph.D. "Question. Persuade. Refer" Booklet. Spokane, WA: QPR Institute, 1995.

3. Carry the Cure's "Committed to Life" Vow. Carry the Cure, November 25, 2020. https://www.youtube.com/watch?v=x-S_bS7FZcA.

Chapter 9 - Boomerang

1. Chapin, Edwin Hubbell, and Josiah H. Gilbert. "Chapter 18." Essay. In Dictionary of Burning Words of Brilliant Writers, 569–69. New York, NY: Wilbur B. Ketcham, 1896.

2. Http://Www.villonfilms.ca/Nelson-Mandela-Prisoner-to-President/. Villon Films, 2012. http://www.villonfilms.ca/nelson-mandela-prisoner-to-president/.

3. Siwa, JoJo. "Jojo Siwa - Boomerang (Official Video) - Youtube." Boomerang (Official Video). JoJo Siwa, May 17, 2016. https://www.youtube.com/watch?v=ypPSrRYOAj4.

4. Warkentin, Sher. "Fun Games for Building Resilience in Children." Fun Games for Building Resilience in Children. Toms of Maine. Accessed September 1, 2021. https://www.tomsofmaine.com/good-matters/healthy-feeling/building-resilience-in-children-using-fungames.

5. Meichenbaum, Donald. Dissertation. HOW EDUCATORS CAN NURTURE RESILIENCE IN HIGH-RISK CHILDREN AND THEIR FAMILIES. Dissertation, The Melissa Institute for Violence Prevention and Treatment, n.d.. http://www.teachsafeschools.org/Resilience.pdf.

6. "How to Build Resiliency." Resilience: Build skills to endure hardship. Mayo Foundation for Medical Education and Research, October 27, 2020. https://www.mayoclinic.org/

testsprocedures/resilience-training/in-depth/resilience/art-20046311.

Chapter 10 - Better Together

1. King, Jr. Martin Luther. 1964. "Learn To Live Together." Recorded at St. Louis, MO. March 22, 1964.

2. Von Schiller, Friedrich. "Theosophy of Julius." Essay. In The Philosophical Letters , edited by Friedrich Von Schiller. Friedrich Von Schiller, 1793. https://www.gutenberg.org/files/6799/6799-h/6799-h.htm.

3. http://www.kiplingsociety.co.uk/poems_lawofjungle.htm

4. Henry, William Writ. "Chapter 8: Union of American Opposition - 1774." Essay. In "Patrick Henry: Life, Correspondences and Speeches 1, 1:193–93. New York, NY: Charles Scribner's Sons, 1891.

5. Wallace, Robert. "Great Day in '76 - July 2, History's Real Story of the Declaration." LIFE, July 6, 1962.

6. Dumas, Alexandre. "The Three Musketeers." Le Siècle , March 1844.

7. Hoefnagels, Anna. "Cree Round Dances." Native Dance RSS, 1 Jan. 2021, https://native-dance.ca/en/renewal/cree-round-dances/.

8. Broken Walls. "2011 Lifelight Festival: Broken Walls." YouTube, 10 Apr. 2012, https://youtu.be/pt-XpZIrTes.

9. Broken Walls. "Circle of the Creator." YouTube, Broken Walls, 9 Aug. 2016, https://youtu.be/ecXynVkWb4k.

10. Broken Walls. "Wave." YouTube, Broken Walls, 30 Aug. 2015, https://youtu.be/YTjTigRBwLI.

APPENDICES

1. Committed to Life Vow
Pagaran, William. "Carry the Cure's 'Committed to Life' Vow." YouTube - Carry the Cure's "Committed to Life" Vow, November 25, 2020. https://youtu.be/x-S_bS7FZcA.

ACKNOWLEDGEMENTS

There are many people who gave me inspiration, help, wisdom, financial support, and encouragement to write this book. I had to learn how to Rise Above all the obstacles that stood in the way of completing it. I am extremely grateful to my friends, family and other Carry the Cure supporters. I'm thankful for all the people I've met along the way, during my many miles traveled to villages, reserves, reservations, towns, cities and communities across the globe. You all have inspired this work. You've also helped me realize the urgency of this resource to help others learn, grow, and rise up.

I do want to highlight a few specific people who were instrumental in seeing this project completed.

First of all, I want to thank my beautiful bride, Amanda Pagaran. You have been my biggest encourager. You helped me believe in myself, my abilities and my talent. You helped me to do things that I thought I could never do. You really helped me to believe what God says in His scriptures, that "I can do all things through Christ who strengthens me." ~ Philippians 4:13. Thank you for your love, kindness and patience. Thanks for the countless hours you spent reading, editing, correcting and discussing creative ideas for *Rise Above It*. This book is as much yours as it is mine. I love you!

I want to say thanks to my mom, Esther Hughes. No matter how tough things got in my childhood, you always helped me believe that tomorrow would be better. You always helped me dream my dreams. I'm living my dreams now because of you.

Thank you, Stephen Knouse, for all your creativity, wisdom, and talents! You made this book flow. You helped it to leap off the page. You masterfully designed this so that anyone could use this book. Thanks for being my long-time friend and ministry partner. Your talents always amaze me!

A huge thanks to Emma Logan for your time, effort and artistry. Thanks for creating photos in such a beautiful way for *Rise Above It*.

A special thanks to Sharon Aubrey of Relevant Publishers LLC. Thanks for sharing your wisdom and insight. Getting this book finished would have been impossible without you.

Thank you, Kris Farmen of Fireweed Editorial for your final edit and suggestions.

Most of all, I'd like to thank Jesus for His never-ending, unfailing love and His amazing grace. You rescued this broken Tlingipino, restored me, redeemed me, and gave me a reason to live. You helped me to forgive others. Most importantly, you taught me to love.

Great News, you can move mountains!

Suicide Peaks Receive New Dena'ina Name of Yuyanq' Ch'ex!

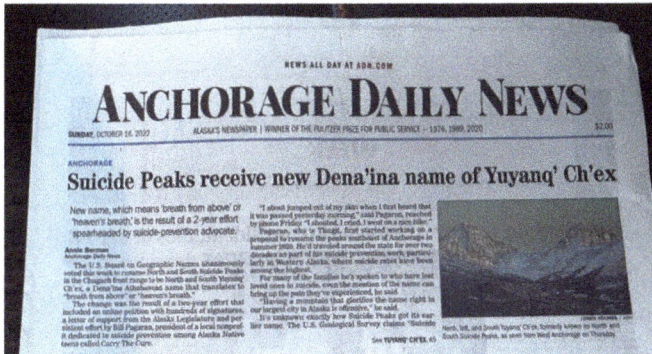

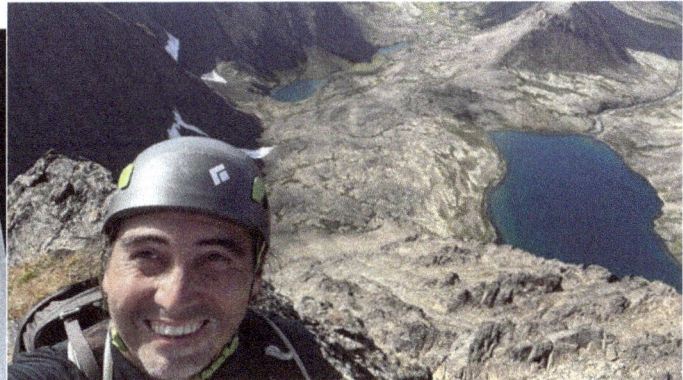

It's official! On October 13, 2022, the US – Board of Geographical Names accepted my proposal to change the name from North and South Suicide Peaks to North and South Yuyanq' Ch'ex.

This name change was a two-and-a-half-year project that began with the suicide awareness hike up South Yuyanq' Ch'ex called **Rise Above It**. Of course, that's what inspired the name of this book.

The change is for real! Thanks to all of you who supported this 2.5-year campaign. Infinite thanks to my wife Amanda Pagaran and my son Reign Pagaran who believed in me the whole time. Special thanks to those who guided me in the application process like Katie Ringsmuth (AK DNR) and Jennifer Runyon (US-BGN). It took hundreds of hours of group zoom calls, personal meetings, phone calls and emails. Thanks to all who gave insight, wisdom and support. Thanks to Anchorage Mayor Bronson, Anchorage Assembly, the Anchorage Federation of Community Councils, Chugach State Park Advisory Board, Friends of Chugach State Park, Alaska Native Corporations, Native Leaders, Dena'ina Linguist Specialists, Shem Pete's Authors (James Kari and Jim Fall), Representative Sarah Vance and the 39 legislators that signed onto a letter of support (just minutes before the US-BGN proposal deadline), Mat-Su Mayor DeVries, Palmer Mayor Carrington, University of Alaska Anchorage, Anchorage School District, First Responders Union, Youth for a Healthier Alaska, Paleontologist/Archeologist Robert King, Vide Kroto, Andrea Ivanoff, Helen Dick, Jon Ross, Dr. Sean Topkok, Crystal Collier, Jennifer Baker, Denali Tshibaka, Niki Tshibaka and so many more.

A special thanks to the Rise Above It hiking team that supported this dream of changing the name of mountains to help others have a hope filled life in Alaska!

The Rise Above It Hiking Team: Douglas Hoffman, Lyon Kopsack, David and Angela Retherford, Fidencio Rodriquez, Austin Skelley, Matt Kratochvil, Tesera and John Moss, NBC American Ninja Warriors Nick Hanson (The Eskimo Ninja) and Jeri D'Aurelio, Marla Rowland, Rev. JD Duncan, Dr. Byron Perkins, Sean Gilbert, Caleb Beauviais, Tshibaka Family, the 7 State of Alaska Commissioners all that attended the opening ceremony for the Rise Above It Hike on August 29, 2020.

Get out and enjoy the mountains! When you visit Anchorage, Alaska visit the Chugach State Park and the newly renamed mountains of North and South Yuyanq' Ch'ex. You can take an easy 4 mile hike to Rabbit Lake to view these beautiful mountains, or dare to summit them. The hike is moderate to difficult. I would start with South Yuyanq' Ch'ex, it's a bit easier. All-Trails App has a great route you can take.

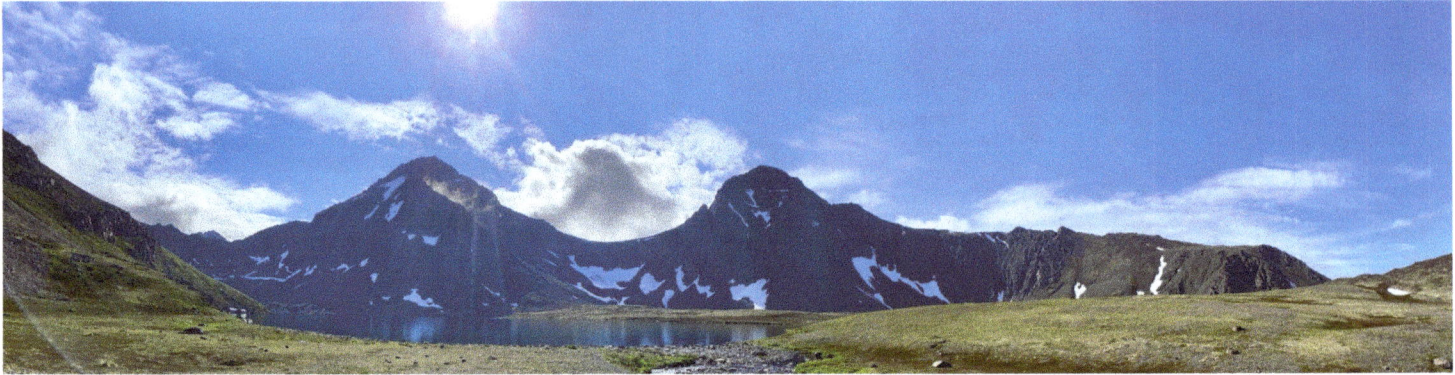

Dena'ina name, Yuyanq' Ch'ex (Heaven's Breath) gifted by Helen Dick and Vide Kroto in 2020. Name change proposal by Bill Pagaran from North and South Suicide Peaks to North and South Yuyanq' Ch'ex officially accepted by the US-Board of Geographical Names October 13, 2022.

This name change was more about highlighting the fact that the people in Alaska and beyond are valuable. Every name matters! Every person matters! There is not mountain that we can't rise above or remove. Take courage for your life's journey and learn to Rise Above the most difficult things you face. The view from the summit is worth the effort to fight for life. Keep climbing, keep rising and keep living.

I've always believed that God can move mountains, but now I have experienced Him moving mountains that I thought would never budge. Each of us have mountains to move in our lives. Speak to your mountains! Believe in your heart that He can remove them, and He will! It doesn't matter if it's a physical, spiritual, financial, or mental mountain; He can remove it. When it's removed, replace it with things full of hope and promise.

www.ingramcontent.com/pod-product-compliance
Lightning Source LLC
Chambersburg PA
CBHW042356030426

42336CB00030B/3497